Living wi ... tation

Dr Keren Fisher qualified in clinical psychology in the 1970s and has a PhD from the University of London. She has worked with orthopaedic and pain patients for the last 30 years and holds a specialist clinical and research appointment in the amputations service in north London as Consultant Clinical Psychologist.

Overcoming Common Problems Series

Selected titles

A full list of titles is available from Sheldon Press,
36 Causton Street, London SW1P 4ST and on our website at
www.sheldonpress.co.uk

Overcoming Common Problems Series

Overcoming Common Problems Series

Overcoming Common Problems

Living with Physical Disability and Amputation

DR KEREN FISHER

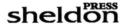

First published in Great Britain in 2009
Sheldon Press
36 Causton Street
London SW1P 4ST

The author and publisher have made every effort to ensure that the
external website and email addresses included in this book are correct and
up to date at the time of going to press. The author and publisher are not
responsible for the content, quality or continuing accessibility of the sites.

British Library Cataloguing-in-Publication Data
A catalogue record for this book is available from the British Library

ISBN 978–1–84709–076–8

1 3 5 7 9 10 8 6 4 2

Typeset by Fakenham Photosetting Ltd, Fakenham, Norfolk
Printed in Great Britain by Ashford Colour Press

Produced on paper from sustainable forests

To our patients who teach us everything useful we know

Contents

Acknowledgements

I must thank my junior colleagues who keep me up to date with new developments and the editorial staff at Sheldon Press for their encouragement and support.

1

Introduction: how can this help me?

This book has its origins in programmes that therapists have developed for people who are trying to cope with disabilities as a result of injuries sustained in accidents or serious illness. Medical treatments naturally take priority in the acute stages but often people are discharged when they are judged well enough to 'live with it'. Little attention used to be paid to the difficulties that 'living with it' may present, and psychological interventions have grown up to help people overcome their barriers to achieving the best possible recovery.

Mood problems such as anxiety, depression and post-traumatic stress disorder commonly accompany life-changing events like serious injury or illness and will interact with the possibility of physical improvement. The chapters that follow look at some ways to deal with these.

The history of the procedures discussed here starts with the behavioural ideas of Dr Fordyce from Seattle in the 1960s. He was the first to suggest that traditional psychological treatment theories based on learning could be applied to managing pain and related disability rather than just mental illness. This breakthrough escalated to the development of pain management programmes in many countries. Learning theory tells us that people carry out behaviours that are rewarded with good outcomes or that avoid bad outcomes. People with disabilities might avoid situations in which they feel anxious, but while they are learning these avoidance tactics they are also limiting their chances of good outcomes. Programmes to help people change these responses allow them to experience a better quality of life.

In the 1970s Dr Aaron Beck contributed the next leap forward by recognizing that people's negative cognitions about failure and helplessness are a major contributor to their emotional distress. Cognitions are thoughts and beliefs that creep into all aspects of emotion and behaviour. Learning to identify and challenge thoughts that don't fit the facts is the essence of cognitive therapy. It allows people to explore their thinking patterns in order to check them with reality and see for themselves whether there is evidence for their beliefs.

By combining the two approaches of learning theory and cognitive challenging, cognitive behaviour therapy (CBT) came into being and flourished for the next 20 or 30 years, becoming the most well-researched and effective treatment for a whole range of physical and mental problems.

While all this was going on, another thread was developing, which had its origins centuries ago in Buddhist practices but which gradually infiltrated 'Western' ideas about management of illness and life in general. This became known as the 'third wave' of CBT. Instead of the emphasis that had previously been placed on the adversarial approach of challenging and rejecting thought content, the new method favoured allowing thoughts and feelings to exist but accepting them as passing mental events. This is now known as acceptance and commitment therapy (ACT). Its main focus is mindfulness – that is, being aware but not being judgemental, paying attention to the present rather than re-living how things were or pre-living how they will be, of accepting how things are rather than attempting to make them different. Mindfulness-based stress management programmes, developed by Dr Kabat-Zinn in Massachusetts, are now beginning to have the same influence as previous CBT-based ones in helping people cope with all kinds of physical and emotional illnesses.

Another aspect of ACT is its emphasis on 'defusion' – that is, examining and preventing the tendency for mere words to dictate emotional and behavioural responses. Words like 'failure', 'stupid' or 'burden' crop up in the language of people who evaluate themselves negatively, and these words then take on meanings that influence how such people view themselves, their world and their future. However, an ACT practitioner will encourage these people to see the words as neutral labels that don't in themselves have the power to cause a response. For example, if I asked you to think about the word 'meng' (my computer reassures me that it doesn't exist), you would probably have little emotional reaction to it. If I then told you it was another word for 'explosion' and gave you the sentence, 'Today, there was a large meng in your neighbour's house,' you would already start to react as if the word had taken on some significance that drives thoughts about danger, safety, loss and insurance. ACT tells us that words are just words and need to be unglued from the emotion we have fused them with.

We are currently at a transitional stage in which the traditional CBT and the modern ACT techniques are becoming integrated, and this book gives you a flavour of both so that you can choose how to deal with any barriers you have to improving your quality of life in spite of your disability.

Probably another of the great challenges following the onset of disability is to rebuild self-esteem in the face of limitation of movement, a decrease in your previous ability, physical scarring and even the loss of limbs. There are many aspects to this, which we will discuss in turn, including recognizing the influence of thinking patterns and learning communication and assertiveness skills in order to improve personal relationships.

Post-traumatic stress disorder occurs after people have experienced or witnessed a life-threatening event. It is accompanied by reliving experiences in flashbacks and nightmares and it is currently a hot topic among the military and families of service personnel. Traditionally the Ministry of Defence in the UK has assumed that the natural bravery and mutual concern for the safety of service personnel have acted to prevent it. However, recent evidence has shown that some members of the forces are more vulnerable than others to this eventuality, and procedures are gradually being developed to enable more timely reporting, diagnosis and treatment of this potentially life-threatening complication. This situation is discussed more fully in Chapter 8.

Goal setting is a central component of rehabilitation and there are golden rules for making sure you keep motivated to achieve your valued activities. Once you have accepted the idea that achieving what you want is still possible while taking your physical state into account, you can keep the process moving forward for as long as you want. A recent survey among people with amputations of their legs showed that most returned to work and about 15 per cent were able to get jobs they actually preferred to the ones they were doing before their accidents. People with long-term pain are also regaining work and improving their lifestyles after following programmes that include an emphasis on goal attainment.

There are special chapters of interest to people with limb loss and related disabilities such as spinal cord injury and brachial plexus avulsion – a situation that occurs when the nerves of the arm are torn out of the spinal cord, leaving the arm paralysed and painful. The experiences of people with problems involving the disconnection of limbs from the spine and the brain are unique in that they involve a mismatch between the brain's actual representation of the body shape and its physical appearance. We shall discuss scientifically tested explanations for phantom limb awareness and pain and a further chapter deals with methods of minimizing the distressing aspects of these by the use of meditation, relaxation and imagery techniques. There is plenty of mythology around these experiences but the book limits itself to practical findings.

The chapters are liberally illustrated with case histories. All the people quoted are fictitious but demonstrate typical examples of the subject under discussion. Their experiences are based on those that actual patients have reported and the techniques used to help their circumstances are those that have been developed in interaction with them, using their feedback to choose the most effective strategies. I hope they will be of interest and use to you too.

2

Understanding the role of thinking in long-term disability

Thoughts, emotions and behaviours

Now that you have to deal with the consequences of your disability you may find that you quite often feel moody, sad, anxious, guilty and frustrated by the limitations it seems to put on your life. Of course these feelings are not universal. If you feel euphoric and full of self-confidence, I don't imagine you will want to read this chapter, or even bother with the book at all, but maybe sometimes when things are not going as well as you would like, you would prefer to regain a better sense of personal control.

To begin with, we could do with knowing more about the process of identifying the thoughts that accompany the emotions that may turn out to limit how you respond to your disability. Figure 2.1 helps to show the processes that the brain goes through to decide how to respond to any new situation. You will notice that the first process happens in the 'Thoughts' box. This in turn determines the 'Emotional response' and, when all aspects of the situation have been added together, the 'Central control' box decides the best way of responding given the information it has received.

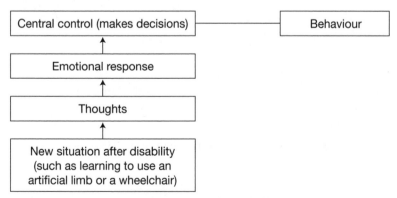

Figure 2.1 Processes that the brain goes through to decide how to respond to a new situation

The plant pot example

As an exercise to begin with, let us imagine the following scene, which will help to illustrate the possible thoughts about an event and the chain of responses that follows from each. Do your best to put yourself in this picture.

You are in the house alone at night. It is very dark and stormy. You hear the wind howling outside and the rain beating on the windows. You have closed the curtains and locked the doors for security. Suddenly in a temporary lull in the storm you hear the plant pots on the front door step fall over. What is your immediate thought?

Your answer may well be one that implies danger. You immediately think, 'There is a burglar or someone trying to break in.' Let us now examine what follows from this thought in terms of the emotional and behavioural responses related to the burglar interpretation (Table 2.1).

Table 2.1 One response to the plant pots falling over

Situation	Plant pots fall over
Thought	It's a burglar
Emotion	Panic, anxiety, fear
Response	Hide, freeze, call police, get a weapon, etc.

These reactions are entirely logical and fit appropriately with the 'it's a burglar' thought. However, there may be other reasons why the plant pots fall over. Maybe you have a pet cat that has been out all day and that you are hoping has come home. Then your thought might be, 'It's Tomcat at last.' The reactions you experience will then fit logically with this thought (Table 2.2).

Table 2.2 Another response to the plant pots falling over

Situation	Plant pots fall over
Thought	It's my Tomcat home at last
Emotion	Pleasure, relief
Response	Get up and let it in

Alternatively you might think, 'There's Tomcat from next door again. He's always digging up my garden.' Then your reactions will be different again (Table 2.3).

Table 2.3 Yet another response to the plant pots falling over

Situation	Plant pots fall over
Thought	It's wretched Tomcat in my garden again
Emotion	Annoyance, irritation
Response	Get up and chase it away

This example illustrates how the interpretation of the situation determines your feelings and responses.

Cognitive fusion

As we have seen, behaviours follow from emotions and emotions follow from thoughts. Thoughts are often experienced in the form of words that represent an actual event (so, the word 'burglar' signifies a dangerous person and a threat to one's safety). A logical pattern falls into place depending on the thought that starts the process. Fearful interpretations lead to anxious emotions, which can be limiting and overwhelming and can lead to loss of coping behaviours. This is an example of cognitive fusion, in which the behaviour (possibly the avoidance of an activity) is 'fused' to the thought that something harmful will happen. We shall return to this in other chapters. After a while fearfulness and lack of a sense of control will lead to depression, which is a whole new problem you can do without.

Thoughts determine behaviour

So, given the situation of chronic disability, thoughts and emotions can influence your behavioural responses and how well you manage your physical limitations. For example, if your friends have moved to a new

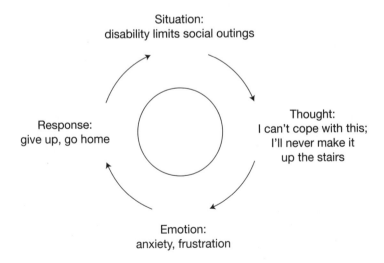

Figure 2.2 **The way in which thoughts determine behaviour**

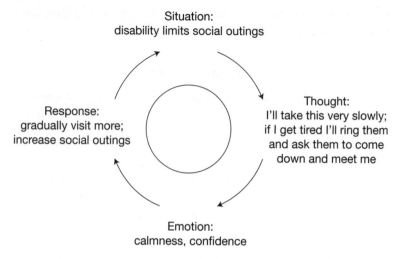

Situation:
disability limits social outings

Response:
gradually visit more;
increase social outings

Thought:
I'll take this very slowly;
if I get tired I'll ring them
and ask them to come
down and meet me

Emotion:
calmness, confidence

Figure 2.3 Alternative problem-solving approach

flat on the first floor of the block you might think in the way shown in Figure 2.2 and risk losing an important friendship. Alternatively, you might interpret the situation with a more problem-solving approach (Figure 2.3) and the disability will become less limiting.

The four aspects of a situation

As we have just been considering, there are usually four parts to any situation.

1 The event itself
2 Your thoughts
3 Your feelings
4 Your behavioural reaction

Most people are only aware of numbers 1 and 3 in this list, but it is your thoughts about the situation that determine how you feel. You need to be able to analyse the meaning you have attached to the event.

The difference between thoughts and emotions

Thoughts are beliefs, images and memories. They may be verbal or visual and will answer the question, 'What was in my mind when I started to feel my mood change?' Feelings are emotions or moods. They can be described in one word and rated for intensity on a scale.

A common scale is 1–100 where 1 is a very low amount of the feeling and 100 is as strong a feeling as you can imagine.

Try the exercise in Table 2.4. Consider whether each item is an emotion or a thought. For each thought, the word 'feel' should be replaced by 'think'.

Table 2.4 Emotions versus thoughts

		Emotion?	Thought?
1	I feel nervous		
2	I feel I'm not going to be able to do this		
3	I feel I'll never again enjoy the things I used to like		
4	I feel something terrible will happen to me		
5	I feel sad		
6	I feel nothing ever goes right now that I have this problem		
7	I feel I'm a failure now		
8	I feel irritated		
9	I feel angry		
10	I feel I can't do even simple things any more		
11	I feel depressed		
12	I feel my friends won't include me in their plans		
13	I feel anxious		
14	I feel I'm a burden on my family		
15	I feel frustrated		
16	I feel I should be quicker or I'll lose my job		
17	I feel guilty		
18	I feel I'm no good for anything any more		
19	I feel panicky		
20	I feel worried		

(Clue: items 1, 5, 8, 9, 11, 13, 15, 17, 19 and 20 are emotions. The others are thoughts.)

Thoughts are probably the easiest part of an event to change. Imagine the situation of being stuck in traffic and whether each factor listed in Table 2.5 would be easy to change.

Table 2.5 Thoughts and emotions when stuck in traffic

		Easy to change? Yes	Easy to change? No
Situation	Stuck in traffic		✓
Thought	This is a disaster	✓	
Emotion	Frustration or panic		✓
Behaviour	Get agitated, shout at other drivers		✓
Alternative	I can listen to the radio while I'm waiting		

It would not be very easy to change the traffic situation and once you have responded to it with a 'disaster' thought then the emotion and behaviour will follow logically from that interpretation. However, if you 'catch' the thought and use an alternative interpretation, then the other aspects will change as well, as we noticed in the plant pot example.

The influence of early experiences

Beliefs about things that influence your quality of life determine how well you cope and how you achieve your personal goals. Beliefs are really assumptions that have been built up over time, often starting in early childhood. Some people have had negative experiences, which lead them to have a low opinion of themselves. Perhaps this has happened to you. When you were very young, an adult or older sibling might have been angry with you because of some problem of their own and might have given you the impression that you were unlovable or lacking in some essential characteristic.

Because you were so young, you believed what was said partly because you didn't have enough language to argue your case and partly because you thought adults must know everything and be right all the time. You stored the unhelpful message in your self-concept and assumed it must be true of you.

Gradually you got on with your life and most of the time you probably managed to succeed in your chosen goals. However, then something bad happened, such as failing an exam, getting divorced or having a serious accident resulting in long-term disability, and the assumption shot to the surface of your mind along with a thought such as, 'Of course this happened to me because I'm such a bad person.' As we have seen, thoughts drive emotions and it's hard to feel ecstatically happy with such a thought about yourself nagging away at your self-confidence. Your mood tends to go down and symptoms of anxiety and depression appear, creating a downward spiral (Figure 2.4).

Early experiences – adults criticize, threaten or bully you

Unhelpful assumptions about your self-concept

Bad life event (such as having a serious injury and disability)

Assumptions reactivated:
'I deserved this, because I'm basically a bad person'

Mood change – symptoms of anxiety or depression

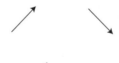

Thoughts, emotion, behaviour

Figure 2.4 Thoughts driving emotions into a downward spiral

The weighty matter of PUDDING thoughts

When things go badly in people's lives, negative thoughts tend to come
to the surface more readily. You might think becoming disabled is an
example of a bad thing happening to you. Negative thoughts might
occur frequently. They appear true and it doesn't occur to you to question them. They appear automatically but they are usually unhelpful
and keep you from moving forward.

This happened to Joshua, who was brought up by a mother with
very low self-esteem. She, of course, had also been raised by a mother
with little parenting skill. Joshua's mother believed that it was bad for
children to feel pleased with their achievements in case they became
'bigheaded' (actually her fear was rather that their success would
make her seem inferior in comparison). Consequently she frequently

told Joshua he wouldn't amount to anything and if he did it would be because he was selfish and careless of other people's feelings. He stored the unhelpful assumption 'I'm a selfish person' in his self-concept.

In fact, Joshua did well at school and later in his job, but at the age of 23 he was an innocent bystander, just walking to the station home from work, when he was caught in crossfire from a gun battle between two teenage boys. He was shot in the leg and ended up ser-iously injured. During his rehabilitation, his physiotherapists tried to encourage him, telling him that he was progressing well, but Joshua didn't seem to respond and seemed quite low in spirits as they tried to stress his improvement. Eventually, he said that he believed he deserved to be shot and became quite distressed. His physiotherapist was astounded and referred him at once for CBT to look at his distorted thoughts.

We shall see in a later chapter how to help you to identify thoughts that may be distorted (that is, thoughts that don't fit the facts very well) and that may be keeping your mood low or anxious. A useful label for these thoughts is PUDDING:

Plausible
Unhelpful
Distorted
Demoralizing
Involuntary
Negative
Groundless

The thoughts are *plausible* because there is often a grain of truth in them. It is often true that you cannot walk so well with an artificial leg as with your two natural ones, or pick things up easily if your hand is paralysed. However, it is *unhelpful* to focus on what you cannot rather than what you can do. Thoughts might be *distorted* ('people won't want to include me in their outings now'), which is *demoralizing* and demo-tivating, so that you give up easily. They are also *involuntary*, and the more downhearted you feel the more *negative* thoughts will occur to you automatically with no apparent effort on your part. It often turns out they are *groundless*, such as your childhood belief that you are a bad person because your mother criticized you for a small offence like breaking a cheap vase by accident. Joshua's belief that personal progress meant selfishness was clearly mistaken.

The good news is that thoughts and beliefs can be changed if we look at the facts and actual outcomes.

If you recognize that you have a lot of PUDDING thoughts like these then you may also notice that you feel more limited by your disability than others in your situation. The next exercise will help you get started on improving your whole quality of life!

Exercise to catch unhelpful thoughts – the ABCD of cognitive therapy

The ABCD of cognitive therapy explains the steps between an event and your response to it.

A: event
C: reaction, but although you may only be aware of these two steps initially, remember
B: interpretation, which fits in between
D: response

To start with you might assume that the event (A) caused the reaction (C) and your response (D) but if you practise stepping back and asking yourself for your thoughts ('What was in my mind when I began to feel my mood change?'), you will soon recognize that the order is really ABCD.

Attempt to catch some unhelpful thoughts about a situation (A) that occur to you in the next few days and jot them down on a mood log form modelled after Table 2.6. You may only be aware of your emotional reaction (C) to the situation to start with, but think about the way you have interpreted it (B). This is really the cause of C. What you did (your behavioural response) is (D) and you will notice that it will fit with whatever your thoughts (B) caused you to feel emotionally (C), just as we found in the plant pot example. However, as you do this exercise, keep realistic – you won't get rid of your disability just by choosing to have positive thoughts!

Table 2.6 A mood log form

Step 1 – Event (A)	Step 2 – Feelings (C)	Step 3 – Thoughts (B)	Step 4 – Behavioural response (D)
Describe the upsetting event	What emotion did you feel? Angry, sad, depressed? How much? (0–100 per cent)	What did you think at the time of this event? What were the actual words you said to yourself?	What did you do?

Did you have any difficulty with this exercise? Many people do, and it quite often takes a lot of practice to disentangle the thoughts from the emotions. However, don't give up, because your effort at getting the hang of it will be well repaid with growing personal control over your life.

Let's look at how some others filled the form in. First let's take Sally's form. She had an above-knee (transfemoral) amputation following a motorcycle accident six months ago and is still trying to get used to walking on her artificial leg. As you can see (Table 2.7), Sally didn't realize that 'I felt that I was stupid' was actually a thought. There are a few clues to what emotions she felt – 'angry', 'guilty' and 'sad'. These were produced by the thoughts that she should have made better progress, that people would assume she was drunk and that she had caused her boyfriend trouble. Perhaps these thoughts are distortions.

Table 2.7 Sally's mood log

Step 1 – Event (A)	Step 2 – Feelings (C)	Step 3 – Thoughts (B)	Step 4 – Behavioural response (D)
Describe the upsetting event	What emotion did you feel? Angry, sad, depressed? How much? (0–100 per cent)	What did you think at the time of this event? What were the actual words you said to yourself?	What did you do?
I fell while trying to walk up the hill near my house	I felt I was stupid and people would think I was drunk. I tried to get up but I couldn't get my balance. I was angry at myself for not making better progress. My boyfriend had to leave work early in the end to come and help me get home and I felt guilty at the trouble I had caused him		I felt stupid and sad. I cried most of the evening

Now let's have a look at what Clive has put on his form (Table 2.8). He injured his neck in a car accident a year ago and has had a chance for more practice at helping himself to gain control of his thoughts of helplessness. He was able to separate his emotions from his thoughts and probably decided his annoyance at the cancellation of the bus was justified, so that didn't affect his self-esteem. He made a plan to walk as best he could, apologize for his lateness and deal with the reaction of his boss when he was faced with it. In fact, it didn't turn out as badly as he expected, so the next time the bus is cancelled he might think, 'My boss is quite understanding when I have to walk' and then he will feel less anxious (though still probably annoyed).

Table 2.8 Clive's mood log

Step 1 – Event (A)	Step 2 – Feelings (C)	Step 3 – Thoughts (B)	Step 4 – Behavioural response (D)
Describe the upsetting event	What emotion did you feel? Angry, sad, depressed? How much? (0–100 per cent)	What did you think at the time of this event? What were the actual words you said to yourself?	What did you do?
The bus was cancelled and I had to walk to work. It is about a mile and takes me a good half an hour	Anxious (70 per cent) Annoyed (50 per cent)	I shall be late for work. My boss will think I don't pull my weight. My early clients will be kept waiting	Walked as best I could and apologized to my boss and my clients – one of whom was late too because of the bus

Sally didn't think she had been helped much by filling in her form and thought she would give it up as a waste of time. However, at her next visit to the orthopaedic clinic she happened to meet Clive and discussed it with him. He helped her fill in another form in a way that enabled her to see how useful it could be (Table 2.9).

These examples may have helped you with your thoughts and emotions. Have another go if you're not satisfied with your first attempt. Or you might prefer to devise your own record form.

Think about things you would like to achieve that perhaps you haven't dared risk for fear of disaster. Jot down your actual thoughts and see if these are causing emotions that are holding you up. Now that you are more familiar with noticing the difference between thoughts and feelings, you might find this easier but still wonder what to do next to bring about change.

Perhaps, having thought about your thoughts, you are already identifying ways in which they are distorted. If you're still not con-

Table 2.9 Sally's second mood log

Step 1 – Event (A)	Step 2 – Feelings (C)	Step 3 – Thoughts (B)	Step 4 – Behavioural response (D)
Describe the upsetting event	What emotion did you feel? Angry, sad, depressed? How much? (0–100 per cent)	What did you think at the time of this event? What were the actual words you said to yourself?	What did you do?
Falling over near my house	Angry (30 per cent) Sad (80 per cent) Guilty (20 per cent)	I am angry that I can't walk as well as I should I am very upset about losing my leg and not being able to walk as well as I used to. I feel pathetic that I'm so dependent I need to get my boyfriend to help me get home	Still felt sad but decided to discuss it with my physiotherapist and practise getting up from the ground alone

vinced, review Sally's and Clive's thoughts to see how they led to the emotions each person experienced and how the thoughts changed with better information – Sally's reduced anger once she decided to ask for the physiotherapist's help and Clive's realization his boss was understanding.

Once you believe you are confident in understanding how your thoughts influence how you feel, you are ready to tackle the next step, which is learning to identify possible distortions in your PUDDING thoughts. This will help you improve your mood and enable you to better achieve your goals. We will look again at Joshua's problem to see how he got on with his CBT.

3

Identifying negative thinking in long-term disability

As we saw in the previous chapter, negative and distorted thoughts can have a harmful effect on how we cope with any new situation. Research shows that negative automatic thoughts are associated with more distress, medication, disability and pain.

Negative feelings (negative emotions) are signals that thoughts need to be checked out. There are many ways in which automatic thoughts can be distorted. Maybe the thoughts are over-generalized and exaggerated, or maybe you are predicting that things will turn out badly without giving yourself the chance to try them out. Maybe you are thinking that not just the consequences of your injury but the whole of your life and your relationships will end in disaster. Focusing on the immediate situation and the way you have interpreted it will help you to regain a sense of self-confidence.

Negative thinking in anxiety

Anxiety is accompanied by a wide range of physical symptoms that are distressing in themselves: rapid breathing, accelerating heart rate, dizziness, nausea, headache, sweating, dryness of mouth, tightening of throat, pain in various sets of muscles and so on. When the state of anxiety is prolonged – that is, chronic – these frightening, uncontrollable symptoms may take the form of what seems to be a real disease or disability.

One of the most important facts you could call to mind at critical moments is that these symptoms are *not* dangerous. None of these physical or emotional reactions indicates that you are dangerously ill or 'going crazy'. They are unpleasant. They are uncomfortable, but they can be tolerated until they go away once you identify the associated thoughts that contribute to your situation.

Sometimes when severely anxious people become intensely aware of their unpleasant physical and emotional reactions, they begin to fear the symptoms themselves even more than the situation that triggers them.

Maria has a spinal injury and is paralysed below the waist. Generally she copes well, but she has recently experienced panic attacks, which make her fearful of going out alone. When she notices her heart pounding, she becomes convinced that she is really ill and her thoughts become ever more focused on the terrible consequences of having a heart attack or stroke. The more upset she becomes, the worse her symptoms feel and she risks getting into a self-perpetuating spiral of increasingly intense emotional and physical suffering.

Negative thinking in post-traumatic stress disorder

Post-traumatic stress disorder (PTSD) is recognized as an anxiety state that can occur in survivors of a wide variety of conditions, including accidents, natural disasters and war. In order to have it diagnosed you must have witnessed or experienced a serious threat to life or physical well-being, then re-experience the event in some way (in thoughts or nightmares) and persistently avoid situations or activities associated with the trauma, or feel numb about it.

Changes in mood are common in PTSD, ranging from anger, shame, guilt, feeling isolated and alone, to a sense of life being pointless, having a diminished interest in the future and experiencing depression. Thoughts and beliefs are characterized by a preoccupation with the traumatic event. Intrusive thoughts and images may keep recurring and cause you to feel as if you were reliving the event. This can take the form of flashbacks, nightmares or hallucinations. Reminders of the event, such as television or newspaper articles, may also trigger these thoughts. Alternatively, there may be difficulty remembering certain parts of the event.

Traumatic events can create panic attacks in a number of situations that have some association with the original incident. They then make you question your basic beliefs about your own safety, and this leads to a sense of being out of control.

Survivors of trauma may feel that their beliefs about themselves and the world are shattered. They might interpret the intrusive thoughts as meaning they are about to go crazy. Accident victims might interpret the intrusions as indicating that they are going to suffer for ever. Some typical thoughts are, 'My life is ruined,' 'Something is seriously wrong with me,' 'I will never get over this,' 'I will not live long,' 'I should not have survived,' 'It's all my fault.'

Omar was injured in a terrorist bombing incident three years ago. He survived, though he had severe injuries including burns to his legs and back. He has been constantly bothered by dreams and flashbacks about the incident. While he is trying to concentrate on other things, he is suddenly back in the street choking with the smoke and he appears to be watching a film with himself as one of the characters inside the picture. Although the bomb attack was years ago, he still experiences the terror and panic as if it only just happened today. This is because he re-experiences living through the event, rather than just remembering it. All the emotional suffering he felt at the time is still part of the intrusive reliving effect.

Nightmares also keep the incident fresh in his mind. They occur most nights and cause him to wake up in a panic. He has to get up and tries to distract himself with other activities until he thinks he can risk returning to bed. He has been unable to make much progress with rehabilitation because he is still so concerned with thoughts and beliefs about the attack and his own inability to help other injured people. Although he has been reassured by his cognitive therapist that his anxiety is normal for someone who has suffered a life-threatening event, he needs to learn techniques to lessen his emotional distress to allow his brain to concentrate on progress in other areas.

Negative thinking in depression

If you are depressed, it is likely that negative thoughts are responsible for your sad feeling. These thoughts tend to be automatic. They are not arrived at on the basis of reason and logic – they just seem to happen. The thoughts are related to the low opinion depressed people have of themselves, rather than to reality. The thoughts are not based on fact and serve no useful purpose. They make you feel worse and they get in the way of achieving what you really want out of life. If you consider them carefully you will probably find that you have jumped to a conclusion that is really not accurate.

Even though thoughts aren't based on fact, they probably seem perfectly believable at the time that you have them. They are usually accepted as reasonable and correct, just like a realistic thought such as, 'it is raining today'. The more people believe these negative thoughts the more negative emotions they feel, so that a downward spiral develops, which makes negative PUDDING thoughts even more frequent.

Most automatic thoughts have a grain of truth in them but are so distorted that they are inaccurate. Distortions are good news because they mean the thought is probably untrue and need not be causing you distress.

Exercise to identify distortions in thoughts

Remember, thoughts are interpretations of events that may be based on previous assumptions that are incorrect. The thoughts in Table 3.1, although they look true and may occur to you frequently, contain misrepresentations that keep your mood low and may prevent the best possible coping response. Identify the distortions in the thoughts in Table 3.1.

Table 3.1 What are the distortions in these thoughts?

Thought
I'm not going to be able to do this
I'll never again enjoy the things I used to like
Terrible things always happen to me
Nothing ever goes right now I have this disability
I'm a failure now
I can't do even simple things any more
My friends won't want to include me in their plans
I'm a burden on my family
I should be quicker or I'll lose my job
I'm no good for anything any more, I'm useless

Checklist of negative automatic thoughts

Below is a list of different types of negative automatic thoughts.

1   Over-generalization. You look at things in absolute, black and white terms with no shades of grey. Words like 'everything', 'nothing', 'always', 'never', 'everyone', 'no one' give this away. *Example*: Everything always goes badly for me. *Alternative*: Some things go badly for me just like anyone else but some things go well.

2   Mental filter. You focus on one negative detail and exclude the more positive overall outcome. *Example*: Not being able to clean the bath means I can't even do simple things. *Alternative*: This is not a simple task for someone with my problem. I can do many other things.

3   Jumping to conclusions. You predict that things will turn out badly with little or no basis. *Example*: If this goes on, I'll end up completely dependent on other people. *Alternative*: That is very unlikely, as I don't know anyone with a problem like mine who can't manage to do things alone.

4 Mind-reading. You assume people are reacting negatively when there's no definite evidence. *Example*: My friends passed me in the street without speaking to me. They must think I'm such bad company that they don't want to bother with me. *Alternative*: No one has said I'm bad company. Maybe they were talking to each other and didn't see me.

5 Catastrophizing. You make the situation out to be much worse than it is. *Example*: This new pain on top of my injury is a complete disaster. Now I can't get on with my life. *Alternative*: I have coped with setbacks before and learned some useful strategies.

6 Labelling. You identify with your shortcomings. *Example*: I did that all wrong. I'm a fool and a loser. *Alternative*: I made a mistake on that occasion.

7 Emotional reasoning. You think something about yourself must be true because you strongly believe it. *Example*: I feel like an idiot, so I really must be one. *Alternative*: What evidence do I have that this is true? Maybe there isn't any such evidence and my feeling (actually my belief) doesn't fit the facts.

8 Personalization and blame. You blame yourself for something you weren't entirely responsible for, or you blame other people and overlook ways in which your own approach might contribute to a problem. *Example*: I always get bad service when I go to my doctor. I must be a nuisance. *Alternative*: My doctor doesn't know everything about my disability. I can't expect a cure when no one knows how to achieve it. Maybe there are some things I can do for myself.

9 'Should' statements. You criticize yourself or other people with 'shoulds' or 'shouldn'ts'. 'Musts', 'ought to's' and 'have to's' are similar offenders. *Example*: I should be able to walk faster than this. *Alternative*: There's no rulebook. I will do the best I can and set realistic goals.

10 Dual standard. You judge yourself by harsher standards than you would your best friends. *Example*: I can't keep up with all my tasks; I'm pathetic. *Alternative*: I wouldn't call my best friend pathetic. I would be sympathetic and offer him or her a break and a drink.

On page 22 is the table of thoughts again with some suggestions about which distortions were present (Table 3.2).

Do you recognize any of these thoughts about yourself that may get in the way of how you cope with your disability? If so, the good news is that they are PUDDING thoughts and can be discarded with a bit more practice so that they stop causing you distress.

Table 3.2 Thoughts and the distortions in them

Thought	Distortion (see text for explanation)
I'm not going to be able to do this	3
I'll never again enjoy the things I used to like	1,3
Terrible things always happen to me	1,5
Nothing ever goes right now I have this disability	1
I'm a failure now	5,7
I can't do even simple things any more	2
My friends won't want to include me in their plans	4
I'm a burden on my family	4,8
I should be quicker or I'll lose my job	9
I'm no good for anything any more, I'm useless	6,7,10

One of the sessions Omar had with his CBT therapist focused on the thoughts he had been having after watching a news report about terrorists abroad, and he was asked to fill in a form similar to the ones in Chapter 2. Note that Omar has also been asked how much he believes his thoughts are true. This helps to record the changes that identifying and challenging the thoughts can make (Table 3.3).

Table 3.3 Omar's mood log

Step 1 – Event (A)	Step 2 – Feelings (C)	Step 3 – Thoughts (B)	Step 4 – Behavioural response (D)
Describe the upsetting event	What emotion did you feel? Angry, sad, depressed? How much? (0–100 per cent)	What did you think at the time of this event? What were the actual words you said to yourself?	What did you do?
Watching news on television about terrorists	Panic (95 per cent) Anxiety (100 per cent) Depression (90 per cent)	I will never get over over it (95 per cent) I feel guilty I survived (80 per cent) I am not safe outside my house (100 per cent) Other people might attack again (95 per cent)	Turn off TV. Play computer games to distract myself. Give up doing my college homework. Sleep badly

These thoughts influence Omar's emotional reaction and his behavioural response so that he is unable to carry out his planned activities for the evening and gets behind with his college assignments. In addition, the thoughts not only relate to Omar's experience of the bomb attack but also include assumptions about other people and his future. His therapist gave him the checklist to help him to understand how his thoughts were distorted, and Omar was able to observe that he was over-generalizing and jumping to conclusions, personalizing and mind-reading. He found this useful in realizing that his emotional reactions need not be so incapacitating, and he soon moved on to the next step of learning to challenge his automatic thoughts.

Core beliefs

Core beliefs or schemas are particularly deeply rooted ideas about your self, your world and your future. They have developed over time and are probably almost as old as you are. They become stronger each time they are triggered by important events in your life. They are thoughts like 'I can't deal with this – I am worthless,' or 'No one will love me.' Distorted schemas produce very unhelpful assumptions. Changing these assumptions involves thinking about your thinking in order to weaken old unhelpful core beliefs and strengthen new ones.

If you have a thought that is often associated with especially strong emotional feelings of anxiety or depression it might reflect a core belief. Try the downward arrow technique to identify what it is – usually a belief reflecting helplessness or unlovableness. Start by writing down the initial thought, which might appear quite trivial to start with. Then ask yourself, 'If that were true, why is it a problem?' This question is represented by a downward arrow. Write down the answer you tell yourself and then add the arrow and ask yourself the question again. Keep going with this procedure until you reach the core belief. You will recognize this as the thought that best fits the strong emotion you experienced with the original thought. It will probably include ideas about being abandoned by important people in your life or being trapped in a disastrous situation that you are incapable of changing.

Joshua, whom we met in Chapter 2, had a core belief in his self-concept that he hadn't been aware of for many years, until he was randomly injured in a gang fight. He was unable to progress with his rehabilitation and told his physiotherapist he wasn't surprised he was shot but he also felt depressed. At an early session of cognitive therapy his therapist tried the downward arrow technique to help identify the nature of his core belief and also to spot PUDDING thoughts along the way. The therapist asked Joshua for an example of a recent situation in which he had felt particularly depressed and then to remember what was in his mind at the time. Joshua reported an instance of his physiotherapist congratulating him for some small improvement. This mismatch between the event (being congratulated) and the response (being depressed) immediately raised the suspicion of a negative core belief below the surface. He reported his thoughts in the list shown in Figure 3.1. Each arrow means, 'If that were true, why is it a problem?'

While it is surprising that feelings of depression are associated with the situation of being congratulated, it makes perfect sense that they are linked with the thoughts about being unlovable and abandoned. By now, however, you will be able to detect Joshua's thought distortions as personalization, mind-reading, 'shoulds' and jumping to conclusions,

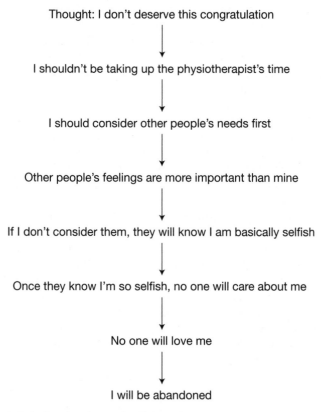

Figure 3.1 Joshua's mismatched thoughts

which have become more obvious as the answers have approached the core belief. Core beliefs are assumptions, not facts, and they can be distorted in the same way as automatic thoughts. They can also be disputed in the same way as PUDDING thoughts, as we shall see in later chapters.

You have now begun the process of testing out negative thoughts, which lead to unhelpful emotions and which may reduce your motivation to change. Don't be discouraged if it seems difficult. What you have learned so far has already helped you to gain more sense of control over your problems.

If you want, you can use a record sheet like the one shown in Table 3.3 but with Step 4 changed so that it records 'Negative interpretations' instead of 'Behavioural response'. You will have had enough practice by now at understanding how emotions can lead to unhelpful activity restrictions. Refer to the checklist on pages 20–1 to identify ways your thoughts might be distorted.

In the next chapter you can find out more about how to consider alternative interpretations and how to challenge negative thoughts in order to prevent the old inevitable pattern of depressed or anxious reactions and restrictive responses.

4

Challenging negative thinking in long-term disability

Having identified the ways in which your thoughts have become distorted, we can now concentrate on looking at the evidence in favour of your interpretation versus the evidence against it. If the evidence is mostly against the thought being true, then the good news is that you can throw it away and concentrate on an interpretation that leads to more positive emotions and responses.

Using cognitive challenges in anxiety

If you feel overwhelmed at the thought of actually confronting an anxiety-triggering situation, look at the thoughts associated with the anxiety and approach the situation gradually. For example, if you are afraid of being knocked over in the street because your injuries mean you can't go fast, you can practise going short distances at a time, first with a friend, then alone until you gain more confidence.

Let's look at an example. Maria, who had panic attacks about going out, spoke to a CBT therapist and between them they identified the thoughts that led to her anxiety:

'I will fall out of the wheelchair and look a fool.'
'I will injure myself and have to go back to hospital.'
'No one will come to help me.'
'My heart beats so fast, I'm sure it will stop.'

So, Maria's thoughts were based on the possibility of being injured falling from her wheelchair and having a heart attack. It is not surprising that she felt anxious and panicky about this, especially since she also thought that people would consider her a fool and not help her.

After discussion with her therapist, however, she realized that her negative thoughts had 'run away with her' and that she probably could have help if she needed it. Maria learned to see that there was a strong PUDDING element in her expectation of going out and it was this that created her panic. She was able to identify distortions as catastrophizing and mind-reading.

Being judge and jury

An important step in dealing with negative unhelpful thoughts is to try to separate the facts in the situation from the negative interpretation you have made. You will remember in the plant pot example (see Chapter 2), the only fact was that the plant pots fell over. There were numerous reasons that you thought of for this, which led to different emotions, some more helpful than others.

It is useful to collect as much evidence as you can to see whether a negative interpretation of an event is the most convincing. For this you could think of yourself as a judge in a court of law, examining the evidence from each side of the argument in turn and then asking the jury to weigh up which is the most likely verdict. Maria filled in a form like the one in Table 4.1.

Maria tried out a strategy of asking her friend to keep behind her in case her belief about falling was true. Then she was able to test out her belief and gain some real evidence to form an alternative view of her ability. She was able to see that even just thinking about the situation

Table 4.1 Maria's thought-challenging worksheet

Situation: Imagining going out alone
Automatic thought: I shall fall out of my wheelchair and no one will help me
How true is it? 70 per cent

What is the evidence for *the thought?*	*What is the evidence* against *the thought?*
I am not always very good at kerbs	I can ask my friend to come with me
I have fallen out several times in the past	I haven't injured myself
When shopping I have to reach up and can overbalance	I can ask other people to reach high shelves for me
	If I don't reach up, I won't overbalance
	People help me every time I've asked

What could be an alternative way of looking at the situation?
No one has said I'm a fool and people do help so it's not a big catastrophe if I fall
How true is the more realistic thought?
People help me if necessary – 90 per cent
How true is your original thought now?
I shall fall out of my wheelchair and no one will help me – 10 per cent

gave her an opportunity to change her catastrophic expectations, and once she had really tried out the task, she had even more evidence that her fear was groundless. She also noticed that her heart rate stayed in a more normal range. We shall return to the problem of increased heart rate in Chapter 8.

Using cognitive challenges in PTSD

Styles of coping with PTSD that try to suppress thoughts about the traumatic event usually lead to more severe symptoms, including more frequent intrusive thoughts. As an experiment, try very hard not to think of a car crash. You will probably notice that however hard you try, not thinking about it is impossible because you have to think about the car crash in order to un-think it.

'Facing up' coping strategies (i.e. trying to deal actively with your reactions) are more profitable in the long run than avoidance coping strategies (distracting yourself or trying to escape from the situation).

Some people learn a system of relaxation exercises to manage severe anxiety, and this is a first step if you have panicky reactions to your intrusive thoughts; alternatively, you may want to look at Chapter 9, on Mindfulness.

Rather than trying to escape from thoughts about the event or distracting yourself by some other activity, you could try holding thoughts, feelings and pictures about the anxiety-producing event in your mind for prolonged periods of time. Mindfulness might also be helpful here.

However, this is very difficult to achieve on your own, and you might want to ask to be referred to a therapist to help you. You will be asked to include as much detail as possible about such things as sights, sounds, smells and feelings to focus on particularly distressing parts of the traumatic event. For instance, you may be asked to stop and repeat yourself and be prompted for more detail. You may be asked to hold or 'freeze' a particular distressing image or scene in your mind, without trying to avoid or 'undo' the accompanying emotional reactions.

Eventually the memory for the event may become hazy and the fear reactions will subside. Some people report feeling 'bored' by trying to remember it. This is a good sign and one that usually leads to a noticeable reduction in intrusive thoughts and dreams.

Eye movement desensitization and reprocessing

Eye movement desensitization and reprocessing (often abbreviated to EMDR) is a relatively new technique, usually needing the help of a trained therapist. It is included here so that you can ask your doctor to refer you if you think it might help you. It appears that repeated eye movements enable the anxiety reaction to an intrusive image to be reduced as the scene is held in imagination. This technique can bring about change in feelings, thoughts and physical sensations of anxiety. Gradually a more positive belief about yourself can take the place of negative thoughts about the event and your difficulties coping with it.

These procedures can lead to permanent changes in the memory of the trauma and to lasting improvement in your feelings. These changes and improvements include no longer being afraid of the circumstances around the event, being able to make a more accurate estimation of the probability of it happening again, and changes in the fear you may have in other situations.

There are no easy solutions to PTSD. You will have discovered that trying to avoid thinking about it does not make it go away. It is better to 'grasp the nettle' and deal with intrusive thoughts so that the traumatic event can be put away as a memory from the past rather than a constantly renewed experience.

Facts and evidence

As an example, let us return to the story of Omar, who was injured in a terrorist bombing. You will remember one of his thoughts was, 'I am not safe outside my house,' but he later identified some distortions such as over-generalization and jumping to conclusions.

The facts were:

- On one occasion there was a terrorist attack.
- Omar had been out of his house safely on countless other occasions.
- The attack was so unusual that the whole country was shocked by it.
- In the three years since the attack there had been no other instances of terrorism anywhere near his neighbourhood.
- Terrorist attacks are still so rare that they are newsworthy and so articles will appear from time to time.

Focusing on the facts could help Omar look at the situation more realistically. He could examine the evidence for and against his thought and then see if he feels better by filling in a table like Maria's (Table 4.2).

Table 4.2 Omar's thought-challenging worksheet

Situation: Watching news on television about terrorists
Automatic thought: I am not safe outside my house
How true is it? 100 per cent

What is the evidence for *the thought?*	*What is the evidence* against *the thought?*
I was injured in an attack	I went out all the time safely before
Terrorism is often in the news	I have often been out since
Terrorism does a lot of damage	I have never been injured again
to people's lives	There has never been another incident here
	It was one isolated, shocking incident

What could be an alternative way of looking at the situation?
I am probably just as safe as I used to be. There is more vigilance against terrorism than there used to be so less chance of it happening again
How true is the more realistic thought?
I am probably just as safe as before – 80 per cent
How true is your original thought now?
I am not safe outside my house – 15 per cent

So Omar has learned that the facts in favour of his alternative thoughts outweigh the evidence for his initial thought. He can now remind himself that it is more likely he will be safe out of doors and maybe he will try and get more evidence by going out more often.

Using cognitive challenges in depression

'No one will care about me.'
'I deserve the bad things that happen to me. People will soon realize how selfish I am.'

These are some of the thoughts Joshua reported which were associated with his depressed feelings in rehabilitation. You will remember his therapist helped him to identify the steps that his thoughts went through on the way to his core belief about being unlovable and abandoned. First there were some 'should' thoughts and then mind-reading and jumping to conclusions. His therapist asked him for alternative reactions to the situations he was thinking about during his physiotherapy sessions.

Therapist: Joshua, let's take the thought, 'I shouldn't take up the physiotherapist's time.' Do you think there is an alternative view here, given that you have been admitted to rehabilitation at this time?

Joshua: I feel that I don't deserve it.

Therapist: That's a thought, not a feeling, and thoughts can be both the cause and the effect of moods. If you feel depressed, you are more likely to have negative thoughts about yourself, which then feed your depression. I see you are now taking some medication that might help you to feel better soon, but in the mean time we can look at the thoughts, and that will also help lift your mood. Can you think of any evidence why you are not entitled to physiotherapy time? Has anyone actually said that you are not?

Joshua: No. I suppose if I'm given the opportunity, I should make the best use of it.

Therapist: There goes a 'should' thought again. I think there is a double-standard automatic thought here as well. If you were talking to your best friend, what might you say to him or her? Would you give your friend such a severe instruction?

Joshua: No. I would tell my friend to try to put in as much effort as he can and be glad of any progress, given the severity of his injury.

Therapist: That sounds much better and quite encouraging. You could try saying that to yourself, rather than giving yourself such a bad time that you dishearten yourself. When you say 'other people's feelings are more important than mine', you are putting yourself down again. What makes you think other people are more important?

Joshua: Other people in the rehabilitation programme are progressing quicker than I am so the physiotherapists are more satisfied with them.

Therapist: Are you sure that is a fact rather than an interpretation as seen through the filter of your depressed mood? As an assignment to help you get to the facts, I would like you to ask the physiotherapists if your progress is going OK or if you need to do anything extra. You could also keep a record for yourself so that you can refer to it and see how things have moved along since you started.

Joshua: I can see that would be a good idea. Maybe I could ask for more exercises to do by myself, and then I wouldn't feel so bad about taking up session time.

Therapist: You could do that and I would like it if you did one more thing as well. When your record shows that you have progressed since your last entry, do you think you could be pleased with yourself in the same way you would congratulate your friend? Once you learn to be more satisfied with your own efforts, you will be less dependent on other people's opinion.

Joshua: My mother used to say that I should think of others' feelings before my own. Did she really mean to discourage me from thinking about myself altogether? It seems she didn't ever want me to be pleased with my achievements, but I'm sure that can't always be best.

Therapist: That is certainly a good place to start your alternative view of yourself. Perhaps your mother had her own reasons for wanting you to consider others first, but that doesn't mean you still have to do what she says now you are an adult. Unfortunately what adults say to children can sometimes damage their self-esteem at a young age. The trick is to realize that, as you grow older, more accurate information comes along, which allows you to update your core beliefs. You just need to make use of it so as to avoid the old outdated (and maybe incorrect) patterns of thinking.

Joshua: I feel more encouraged to look at my other automatic thoughts now to see if they could be challenged in the same way.

Therapist: Have a go at filling in this form (Table 4.3) and we can have a look at it next time.

Table 4.3 Joshua's thought-challenging worksheet

Situation: Thinking about my injury
Automatic thought: I deserve the bad things that happen to me
How true is it? 90 per cent

What is the evidence for *the thought?*	*What is the evidence* against *the thought?*
I was the one who got injured	I just happened to be there at the time
Other people get over their injuries	Other people's injuries are less severe
I have worse luck than other people	Other people sometimes have bad luck
I am selfish to think that I need help	I need to prioritize my own progress
	I deserve to progress if I work hard

What could be an alternative way of looking at the situation?
I am jumping to conclusions and assuming I deserve worse things than other people. I can ask to do more for myself between sessions and be more pleased with my progress. I wasn't responsible for my injury but that doesn't mean I deserve only bad things. I can be responsible for my recovery and deserve some good things too
How true is the more realistic thought?
I deserve to progress if I work hard – 75 per cent
How true is your original thought now?
I deserve the bad things that happen to me – 10 per cent

Joshua has made a lot of progress already by weighing up the evidence for and against his automatic thoughts. Unfortunately, he has some deep-rooted core beliefs that he will need to work on for a while yet,

Table 4.4 Maria's combined mood log

Step	Comments
Step 1 – Event Describe the upsetting event	Imagining going out alone
Step 2 – Feelings What emotion did you feel? (Angry, sad, depressed…) How much? (0–100 per cent)	Anxious (80 per cent) Panicky (80 per cent)
Step 3 – Thoughts What did you think at the time of this event? How true would you rate these thoughts (0–100 per cent)?	I will fall out of the wheelchair and look a fool (70 per cent) I will injure myself and have to go back to hospital (100 per cent) No one will come to help me (70 per cent) I will have a heart attack (60 per cent)
Step 4 – Negative interpretation See checklist on pp. 20–1 and record the number (or numbers) of the interpretations that apply to your thoughts	3, 6, 7, 4, 5
Step 5 – Realistic responses What is the evidence? Substitute more realistic thoughts. How true are they?	People have helped me in the past (100 per cent) I have not injured myself (100 per cent) Falling out of the wheelchair doesn't mean that I am a fool (80 per cent) I have not had a heart attack before when I've felt like this (100 per cent)
Step 6 – Outcomes How true are your thoughts from Step 3 now (0–100 per cent)?	I will fall out of the wheelchair and look a fool (10 per cent) I will injure myself and have to go back to hospital (0 per cent) No one will come to help me (0 per cent) I will have a heart attack (0 per cent)
Step 7 – Feelings How bad are your emotions from Step 2 now (0–100 per cent)?	Anxious (40 per cent) Panicky (20 per cent)

but he has learned some of the basic techniques that will continue to help him along.

Maybe you can think of alternative thoughts to a particular negative one that pops up regularly, and this will give you plenty of opportunity to use your new skill. Use a form like the ones in Table 4.1, 4.2 and 4.3.

We can now put all the information together and complete a new mood log that will allow us to chart changes in feelings as well as thoughts. Table 4.4 shows one that Maria filled in. You can devise one for yourself if you like.

5

Body image and self-esteem in long-term disability

What is body image?

Your body image is a mental picture of your own body, which develops very early in life. Part of the picture is made up of physical experiences (what my body feels like) and social experiences (how others behave towards me). Physical appearance is created by individual people in response to the norms that are fashionable in any given culture and time. Many people try to make their bodies conform to their perceived norm, and in the developed world a huge amount of money is spent on diet aids to achieve this. Even so, a few years ago a survey in the USA of 200 non-disabled people found 25 per cent of men and 35 per cent of women had a negative view of their physical attractiveness and, perhaps more surprisingly, more than 85 per cent of them thought that this was more important than fitness and health.

Of course, attractiveness is 'in the eye of the beholder', and not only do we attempt to conform to fashion, but we will alter our view of ourselves depending on the social context. After the survey mentioned above had been completed, a further experiment was carried out to test how consistent satisfaction with body image was in different circumstances. One hundred and seventy-four people (mostly women) filled in a questionnaire about their body image 'at this very moment'. The questionnaire consisted of items about general physical appearance, body size, and shape, weight and attractiveness. Each item could be rated anywhere from 'extremely dissatisfied' to 'extremely satisfied'. Then the respondents were asked to imagine how they would feel in different scenarios – in a bathing costume at a beach party, looking at a fashion magazine, being complimented at an evening party, or finding a pleasing result when weighing themselves. They had to rate themselves again on the satisfaction scale.

When they imagined the beach or fashion magazine situation, the respondents rated their satisfaction lower than they had when considering 'this very moment', and when they imagined the compliments and weight situations they rated their satisfaction higher. So we can't say that body image is one thing, but it appears to depend on moment-to-moment appraisal in different contexts.

Loss of identity as an effect of changed body image

If your self-image is dependent on your intellectual skills – say an ability to write poetry – then your physical body image might not be so important. However, if your self-image depends on a physical function – say you're very good at dancing – and if that is changed by the disability, then your self-image needs to try to adjust to the new body image.

Alex was an excellent runner. This skill was very important to him since all his life he had the impression that his parents preferred his sister and valued her achievements more than his. Not only did running help him to feel good about himself and his fit, healthy body, but also he knew this was an area that earned him more approval than his sister. Whenever he felt angry, disappointed or sad, he could take to the running track and compensate for his negative emotions with a sense of real well-being.

Unfortunately, he was involved in a serious road accident and suffered many fractures. He was never able to run to his previous ability again and found it too frustrating to settle for a gentle jog, so he gave up altogether.

His self-image had been closely defined by his athletic body and he began to experience the emotional effects of criticisms he had overheard as a child about disability, illness, fitness, unattractiveness and dependence. Since he had previously experienced himself as able to avoid these criticisms by the very skill that he had now lost, he needed to find other ways of confronting these possible insults. The inconsistency between his altered physical agility and his previous perception of his body produced a very difficult emotional tension, and he became quite depressed. His disturbed self-image developed as a result of the need for a new interaction between different expectations, his previous personality characteristics and his more limited physical abilities.

The tension need not be as negative as Alex's experience, though, and will depend on the personal history each individual person brings to the event. Some researchers say it is easier for younger people to adapt as they have a more 'fluid' body image as their bodies mature. Others say older people can adapt more easily because they are used to adjusting to age-related change. As with everything else, there is no universal answer. The good news is that most researchers agree there is no strong relationship between the degree of physical disability and emotional adjustment. The key is how you *perceive* the change, and this is determined by your personal thoughts and beliefs, which we will look at in more detail later.

When people become self-conscious about their image, they can have difficulty in all kinds of social interactions. They may be extra-sensitive to any sign of disapproval, and they can become so preoccupied with their appearance and the possibility of criticism that they become distracted and self-absorbed. They don't properly listen to the people they are talking to and this can eventually result in actual (as opposed to perceived) criticism. Other people's reactions towards us are a direct result of how they perceive us to behave towards them. If, since your disability, you're constantly preoccupied by physical problems like the shape of your body, your social interactions might be awkward and limited. If you learn to perceive your body as only a small part of your general social self, then a cascade of emotional and behavioural changes will follow that will lead to more positive social feedback, which in itself will then improve self-esteem.

Would a television makeover help?

Television programmes about improving physical characteristics show glowing self-confident people at the end. How has this been achieved? I guess only through behind-the-scenes work on the relationship between physical appearance and core beliefs about the self. After cosmetic surgery, psychological changes including emotional, perceptual and cognitive changes around body image change are gradual. Surgery in itself does not necessarily lead to positive changes in people's social lives. Television makeovers might help begin the process, but perhaps the cycle can begin in a different place – remember this is all about individual appraisal.

Some television programmes have focused on taking people as they are (it's cheaper for one thing) and encouraging them to try experimenting with situations that they previously avoided. Positive feedback from friends and the public at large have the same effect of enhancing self-confidence and can result in more positive self-esteem than actual body change. Simple adjustments to posture, hairstyle and clothing colours may be the starting point for increased behavioural interaction with others.

Sheena was hurt in a skiing accident, and as well as suffering pain from her injuries she had a bad scar on her face. A plastic surgeon removed it successfully, but Sheena reported that she did not feel any better. Her confidence in social relationships had reduced since her accident, and the surgery had not helped this at all. She needed to look at whether her preoccupation with her appearance had led her to avoid seeing the very people who could encourage her to see herself as just as useful and worthwhile as before.

What is self-esteem?

We have seen that body image is only a part of the way we present ourselves to others. Our self-image is also largely determined by what we think about ourselves and therefore our relationships with other people. Thoughts determine emotions and behaviour, as we saw in Chapter 2. Self-esteem is best described as people's ability to evaluate themselves as worthwhile and deserving of some happiness. It is sometimes thought of as a basic human need and involves respect from others and respect for oneself. People with low self-esteem who do not have much respect for themselves or expect much from others may experience a number of different emotional problems and may seek to compensate themselves in ways that lead to more problems than ever – such as misusing drugs or alcohol. A further problem arises when these people try to decide where their attributes fall short of those that they consider ideal.

Who is ideal?

If you think your body image and thus your self-esteem have deteriorated since your disability, you may think you are further than ever away from your ideal. Perhaps you were always displeased with your appearance and lacked social confidence, and now these aspects seem even less satisfactory than before.

Anne has arthritis and has become less active as her disability and pain have developed. Even as a much younger person she wished she was more attractive and outgoing and now she thinks she might as well give up and settle for being isolated with few friends. She often has the thought, 'If only I were more like Una, I could manage my disability better because I would have more friends. People would still enjoy my company because, if I were like Una, I would be good at witty conversation and could give entertaining dinner parties.'

So Anne values Una because she's witty and entertaining. Anne also knows that Una's husband left her because he preferred less of a social life and longed for a more private and intimate relationship. Anne has compared herself with only those aspects of Una that she thinks she lacks herself. She has idealized those characteristics and decided to discount Una's disadvantages. Una is more witty than Anne but Anne is more loyal and helpful than Una.

Exploring the problem of rating real versus ideal

Maybe you think rank and privilege give people a high score on the 'ideal' scale – royal families, perhaps? Many people with more republican ideas would disagree. Rank and privilege might be good things but they can set people apart and prevent normal social interaction. Therefore, overall they might have a low score.

What about television celebrities? They may have fame and fortune (high scores) but they often have very difficult private and social lives (low scores).

What about your neighbours three doors away? They might be taller, more beautiful people than you but maybe you believe in better discipline for your children and in keeping your house better maintained.

So, we have looked at a number of attributes – wit, wealth, fame and attractiveness – and discovered that none of these make up an ideal person. You already have all the characteristics that you need to feel good about yourself, but perhaps you don't seem to be successful. Your task is to recognize some of your less helpful core beliefs and to learn to identify the self-talk that prevents you appreciating the skills you have.

Effect of physical changes

Maybe not all the changes that you think have occurred since the onset of your disability have been negative. Some people think of themselves as more patient and sympathetic than they were before.

What changes do you think you have experienced since the onset of your disability? Jot down a few ideas in a list of 'good' and 'bad' things.

Other people have done this exercise and here is a list of some possible ways in which they think of themselves with and without their disability:

- physically attractive
- witty
- entertaining
- helpful
- loyal
- confident
- limited
- boring
- sympathetic.

Have a look at the list and add any characteristics from the lists that you have just jotted down that you think are missing and that apply to you. Give each a score out of 100. You could then make two graphs,

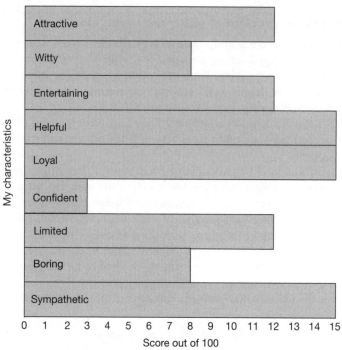

Figure 5.1 Anne's list before her disability

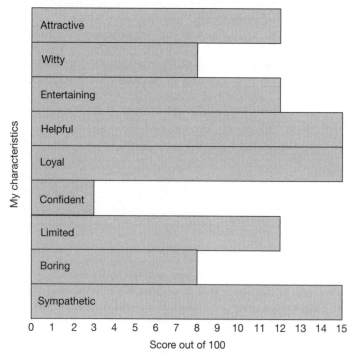

Figure 5.2 Anne's list now, with her disability

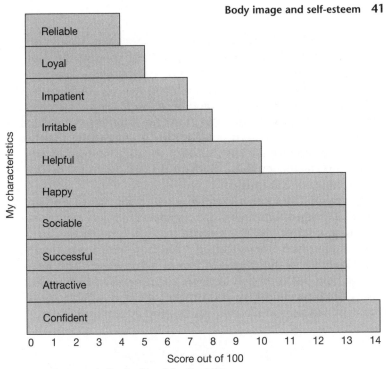

Figure 5.3 Leroy's list before his disability

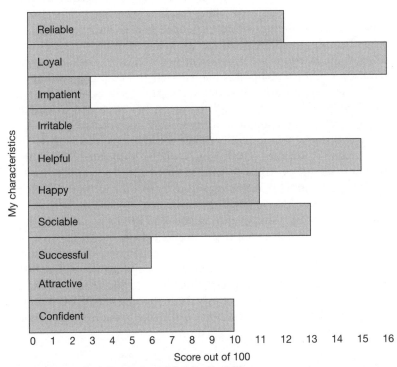

Figure 5.4 Leroy's list now, with his disability

one labelled 'Myself before disability' and one labelled 'Myself now', to see the contrast between your previous self and yourself now. How do the graphs compare?

When Anne did this exercise, she found that the 'building blocks' that made up her 'before' and 'after' selves were identical (Figures 5.1 and 5.2). So Anne has learned that in fact her arthritis has not changed her basic personality. She is no less attractive or entertaining than before (she never considered she was), but she's no less helpful or sympathetic either. She can build on those strengths that she values to improve her social confidence if she wishes.

We can look at another example where more change does appear to have happened. Leroy, who had a spinal cord injury from a mountaineering accident, did this exercise too. His two graphs were a bit different from each other (Figures 5.3 and 5.4). Leroy has learned skills to compensate for his perceived loss of attractiveness and financial success. He is just as sociable as before and now values helpfulness and loyalty. He is less impatient and irritable but more reliable. He is less confident, but he is working on building self-esteem in this area.

Guilt, shame and anger

People who acquire a disability may believe they have become a burden to others and feel guilty for taking up their time. They may also feel ashamed of the abilities of their changed bodies and they might feel angry because things are no longer as they used to be.

All these reactions are normal but not necessary. They are ways of reducing your own ability to value yourself and keep you stuck in low self-esteem. Typical thoughts that accompany feelings of guilt are like Sally's when she thought of having to get her boyfriend to help her home: 'I felt stupid and guilty at the trouble I had caused him.'

Typical shame thoughts are, 'People will think I am too needy. They will be able to see how selfish I am. I will be humiliated.' If you have thoughts like these, you will tend to avoid social encounters for fear of doing something that you regard as shameful and that will expose your basic defects. You might feel ashamed of needing help in the supermarket or of falling over in public. You will be afraid that others' reactions will reinforce your negative core beliefs.

Anger is related to shame – you may blame others for making you feel humiliated. Angry thoughts may well come to the surface more readily than before because everything seems to take more trouble and is more frustrating than previously. Your thought might be, 'He's not doing what I say because he doesn't really care about me.' Your behavioural response may then be to shout at the person who is trying to help. You didn't realize that the thought, 'He doesn't care about me' was *your* thought based on your appreciation of yourself, which you have 'projected' into the other person's mind and attributed to him or her quite by mistake.

The problem of control

Sometimes your new view of yourself is threatened by your apparent loss of control over your previous life. Maybe you were always a 'control freak', and a sense of losing control is very anxiety-producing. You may feel scared, especially in the early days of adjustment, that you will be for ever more a passive receiver of what other people think is good for you. There may be areas in your life, such as being able to make your own decisions or knowing the whereabouts of your children, where a sense of control is paramount in maintaining good self-esteem. Gradually you may notice you have control in the areas you particularly value and you may decide to delegate the rest – maybe trying to control whose turn it was to do the washing up was never worthwhile in the first place. However, if you think your family didn't respect your rota because they didn't respect you as a person, you might need to examine how closely your need for control was an apparent automatic thought that related to some hidden core belief in your actual self-worth.

The highly influential Dr Aaron Beck (the 'father' of CBT) has noted that there are three levels to thinking processes:

1 Automatic thoughts and images
2 Intermediate beliefs – conditional beliefs
3 Core beliefs or schemas.

A schema is a mental representation of our 'self' in the world that serves to filter and organize the information we receive from our senses.

You can think of these three aspects as relating to parts of a boat.

1 The sails of the boat (automatic thoughts) are easy to access and they respond to changes in your day-to-day environment. The wind changing the direction of the sails is like your fluctuations in self-esteem, which depend on feedback from other people (or imagining yourself at a beach party). They are thoughts like, 'I don't feel up to going to that party – people will notice me and I will be embarrassed.'
2 The hull of the boat is like your intermediate or conditional beliefs. They respond more slowly to the tide of change. They are thoughts like '*If* I can't learn to walk better, I can't achieve anything.'

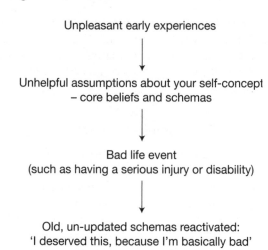

Unpleasant early experiences

Unhelpful assumptions about your self-concept
– core beliefs and schemas

Bad life event
(such as having a serious injury or disability)

Old, un-updated schemas reactivated:
'I deserved this, because I'm basically bad'

Figure 5.5 Critical incidents triggering schema beliefs

3 Core beliefs (see Chapter 3) are like the anchor that keeps the boat of your 'self' in the same place.

Critical incidents can trigger schema beliefs, as we saw in Chapter 3 (Figure 5.5). Getting at core beliefs is a difficult and challenging process. If you think your disability has uncovered some really negative assumptions that you have been carrying around about yourself, you may need to ask your doctor to refer you for CBT. This will help you to identify where your presumed evidence has misled you. However, there's plenty you can do for yourself. Chapter 3 outlines common thinking errors which apply to core beliefs as well as automatic PUDDING thoughts.

Of course, your anchor might be keeping you in a safe haven and your core beliefs might be really useful thoughts instead, such as, 'I can overcome this because I'm basically a capable person who has faced difficult challenges before and survived.'

Alex and Sheena both needed help from a CBT therapist and undertook some of the exercises we have looked at in other chapters to help to improve their core beliefs and self-esteem.

Examine your self-talk

What we say to ourselves – our private internal dialogue that goes on constantly inside our heads – reflects our thoughts. If we have an

Table 5.1 Examples of thoughts, emotions and behaviour that might occur in low self-esteem and good self-esteem

	Low self-esteem		Good self-esteem
Thought	I'm no good at keeping friends; no one likes me	My friend doesn't understand my situation	Here's a chance to learn something about myself; I'll ask for more info
Emotion	Sad, anxious	Angry, frustrated	Motivated, alert
Behaviour	Give up; withdraw from social events	Argue with friend, lose friendship	Get more feedback; learn new ways of relating to people

internal 'parent' who criticizes and punishes us, our thoughts will be largely of low self-worth. Thoughts determine emotions and behaviour. Therefore self-talk influences our thoughts and can determine self-esteem.

Can you identify self-talk that is keeping your self-esteem low? Examples might include:

- I am overwhelmed by my problems.
- I can't achieve what I want.
- I am not very interesting any more.
- I don't meet other people's expectations.
- No one will be interested in me with this pain and disability.

Perhaps you recognized some of those self-statements or you can supply your own.

Let's try an exercise with a situation of a friend who says to you, 'You don't seem to be very bright and breezy these days.' You can respond in ways that reinforce your friend's opinion and reduce your self-esteem, or you can take another view. Whatever self-esteem thoughts you have in response to your friend's remark, matching emotions and behaviours will follow. A few examples are shown in Table 5.1.

Learn about self-acceptance

The 'self' is complex, and since as we have seen, some aspects are more changeable than others, it is never 'one thing'. Therefore feeling good about yourself, or at least accepting your 'self', cannot happen perfectly all the time. There will always be occasions when you would have liked to have behaved differently, received better appreciation of your efforts or been more helpful to someone who asked your advice. This doesn't mean that you are a failure in a global sense, but only that sometimes parts of your 'self' are more successful than others. This is known as the human condition! Given that you're a paid up member of the human race, just like royalty, celebrities or your neighbours three doors away, it follows you will inevitably make some mistakes, misjudge a situation or run out of patience. Giving yourself the label 'failure' is an obvious example of an over-generalization distortion in your thinking. You can revise the exercises in Chapters 3 and 4. If you catch yourself negatively and globally labelling your 'self' you can remind yourself that the particular situation that triggered the thought was probably only one, and there are many others that have shown that you can be successful.

Gary, who had a motorcycle accident and now has a paralysed and painful arm, used to label his 'self' as useless because his disability prevented him playing squash and he lost contact with his club mates. When he finished with rehabilitation and returned to full-time work, he found it easier to change his thought, 'I am a failure' into a self-acceptance thought, 'I would like to play squash like I did before, but as that's not going to happen, I shall brush up my chess instead and join a new club. I might be a failure as a squash player now, but I'm a successful person, capable of change.'

Be on the look out for thoughts that keep you in the same old rut.

Be prepared to try new things or new ways of achieving previous ones. Set yourself new goals that take account of your disability rather than blaming yourself for not achieving your old ones. Have a look at the next chapter on the golden rules of goals.

Self-talk that increases self-esteem uses statements such as:

- I am quite a good ...
- I can usually ...
- I am a survivor because ...

Encourage better self-esteem by:

- discarding failure self-talk;
- setting realistic goals; and
- congratulating yourself for achieving them.

6

Goal setting in long-term disability: the golden rules

Having accepted that you have a disability that no one knows how to cure, one of the first steps you need to take is to get a clear picture of things that you actually want to change, what activities you are interested in doing that would improve your life, and what you need to increase in order to achieve them. These need to be *your* preferences and they need to be important enough to you to keep you progressing even through bad times. You may have been waiting for your strength to improve before you can commit yourself to taking a course such as word processing, French for beginners or an Open University degree. Or you may have decided that when you get better you will be able to visit your elderly parents who live abroad, or get married, or look for a new job. Putting off these achievements means your life is passing by and opportunities are being missed and still your disability hasn't gone away.

You may have noticed that some of these changes have happened as a result of your disability:

1 Reduced
   (a) Work and house work
   (b) Enjoyable activities
   (c) Social activities
2 Increased
   (a) Conflict with family members and friends
   (b) Sleep disturbance
   (c) Rest during the day
   (d) Boredom
   (e) Irritability
   (f) Anxiety and mood problems

You might need a definite change in your lifestyle, one that allows you to take up new fulfilling activities within your physical limitations in a gradual and determined way, in order to compensate for those that you cannot any longer pursue.

Golden rule 1 – choosing the right goals

Goals are actions to be achieved, which are easy to observe and measure and which are particularly important in your life. They let you take control. They allow problem areas to be broken down into manageable bits – bits that give focus and structure to a big problem situation, such as life with a long-term disability – and enable you to test out any assumptions that you have about your capability.

Goals increase self-esteem – if self-esteem is high you are more likely to work at your best. Goal achievement is highest when the goals that are set are moderately difficult rather than too easy or too tough. If they are too easy they will not give a sense of achievement, and if they are too difficult they will cause anxiety, frustration and a sense of failure – both will reduce your motivation. Also, goals give knowledge and feedback about thoughts and other barriers that prevent you achieving them, and they inform you how to set up the goal for better success next time. Most realistic goals can be achieved by working at them slowly and steadily. If you aren't achieving in one area, it's probably not an important enough goal.

You may have come across the description SMART before. The letters stand for these aspects of goal setting:

- Specific – to help you have a clear focus. If you choose a problem area such as 'getting fitter' this is not defined specifically enough to know when you have achieved progress. Define the goal in terms of a specific activity, for example, 'going swimming'.
  Measurable – to identify the amount achieved, for example, a number of lengths of the local pool.
  Achievable – to enable planning and prioritizing. Decide how much of the goal you are likely to achieve given other demands on your life, for example, four lengths a week.
  Realistic – to be appropriate to your lifestyle, age and physical ability. Choose goals that take account of the energy, money and time you can afford to spend.
  Timed – to allow you to plan how much you can progress in the time available. Agree with a friend when to give an account of your progress, for example, 12 lengths by the end of the month.

Let's look at how Joshua started on this aspect of dealing with his low mood and motivation. He discussed the problem of meeting new friends with his CBT therapist.

Joshua: I don't know how to set about meeting new people.

Therapist: What hobbies are you interested in?

Joshua: I used to like art.

Therapist: Do you think there might be a class near where you live?

Joshua: I don't know but I could find out from the library.

Therapist: That's a good idea. We can put that on your goal form this week. I notice the physiotherapists are asking you to increase your walking too. Goals are easier to achieve if they are linked to a valuable activity in your life. Walking with your damaged leg is difficult to do every day just for itself. You will achieve this goal better if it enables something you want to do it for – increase the time you can walk to get to the shops, get to the pub or visit a friend.

Joshua: Being able to get to the pub would be good. Then I can meet my friends there too.

Therapist: We'll put both those goals on the form then. I'll show you how the goal form works a bit later.

You might want to involve others in deciding what goals to prioritize. Family negotiation is important if you want to regain independence and not seem to push away those people who have been caring for you. On the other hand, try not to choose goals that depend on someone else doing something to help. You may find they are not willing or available and this will hold you up. See what you can do on your own.

Choose a variety of tasks that involve different positions of the body so some parts rest while others are active.

Golden rule 2 – pacing

Look at what is required in what you want to achieve. If you want to take on some work in the home or for charity, break down what this will entail into how much walking, sitting or reading this requires and set yourself targets to increase little by little each week. Make sure your targets are small enough for you to succeed at them and stick to the amount you have decided on. Do not exceed a target just because you feel a bit better. Overdoing things on a good day and spending the next three days in bed gradually reduces your tolerance. Building up slowly and setting targets that you can achieve even on bad days gradually increases your tolerance. Use breaks to practise relaxation or meditation to restore your energy and reduce any discomfort. Prioritize jobs that have to be done but rest between chores. Beware of the roller coaster.

Anil had a serious back injury from a fall from scaffolding. He could do only small amounts of activity at a time but tried to use days when he felt better to catch up on his DIY projects, and on one occasion he spent three hours in awkward positions fixing the plumbing in his new bathroom. After this, he was bothered by so much pain and stiffness that he needed to stay in bed for two days, which undermined the fitness he had previously achieved with regular exercises. When he went back to his plumbing goal, he was weaker than before and he was anxious about increasing his discomfort again. He achieved only about one hour's worth of work, felt even worse and retired to bed for the rest of the week, not only in pain but also depressed at his setback.

Fortunately, Anil soon had a follow-up appointment with his CBT therapist who helped him set his pacing targets and explained that he needed to take frequent short breaks. If after 20 minutes at his plumbing, he was exhausted for the rest of the day, he needed to reduce this to 15 minutes. If this still exhausted him he could reduce it to 10 minutes. He could then take a 15-minute break before doing another 10 minutes. This way he would be able to continue his plumbing

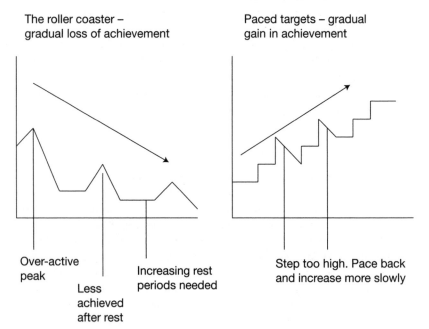

The roller coaster –
gradual loss of achievement

Paced targets – gradual
gain in achievement

Over-active
peak

Less
achieved
after rest

Increasing rest
periods needed

Step too high. Pace back
and increase more slowly

Figure 6.1 The need for pacing

project the next day instead of needing several days' rest to overcome the effects of an overdose of one activity.

Then he could gradually increase. He could pace up every three days or so. He could build up his targets slowly – say one minute at a time. If that was successful for three or more consecutive increases, he could afford to be a bit more ambitious – perhaps he could increase by three minutes at a time. If that seemed too much, he would need to pace back to a two minute increase (Figure 6.1).

So Anil learned the rules for pacing targets. You can benefit from his experience if this is all too familiar to you. Stick to your targets as much as possible – giving up because it's a bad day and then trying to catch up on a better day will get you back on the roller coaster.

Golden rule 3 – keeping records

Joshua's therapist showed him a form called a goal sheet (Table 6.1) and discussed what should go in each section. The point of this scaling is to give a clear picture of how much of the goal can be reasonably achieved and then to keep a record with a score that indicates how well you actually did in the time available.

Table 6.1 The goal sheet

Score	Goal number 1	Goal number 2	Goal number 3	Goal number 4
–2: least possible outcome				
–1: what you can do now				
0: expected level				
+1: better than expected				
+2: best possible outcome				
Review date:				

Therapist: Joshua, you decided on two goals, which we can divide up into the bits on the form. First we must decide how much time you want before you review your progress. I suggest a week. Is that OK? Next you can tell me what you can do now about finding out about art classes.

Joshua: I can walk as far as the library.

Therapist: So that's what goes in the section marked –1. If you do less than this, that will go in –2. This section often contains 'Do nothing'. If you stick at –2, this is not an important goal for you. You may have to scrap it and choose something you feel more enthusiastic about. For now, let's carry on. Next you decide what you think is a realistic extra step to achieve in one week.

Joshua: I can get the leaflet about classes, ring around and try and get registered.

Therapist: That seems a lot for just one week. I think getting registered is the best possible outcome and needs to go in the +2 section. All that is really realistic is probably getting the leaflet. That will go in the 0 section. Between those we could put getting the information from ringing the various centres in section +1.

Joshua: So, depending how much I get done, I get a score between –2 and +2 for each goal.

Therapist: That's how it works. Now we have completed that goal and can do the same with your walking one. For this to work properly we need to specify –2, –1, 0, +1, +2 for every goal and not leave any levels blank. Also, we should not leave gaps between levels like saying –1 is 'walk 10 minutes' and 0 is 'walk 15 minutes'. Then you will not be able to score an achievement between 11 and 14 minutes, so the 0 section should include these steps. How many minutes will it take for you to walk to the pub?

Joshua: About 15 I think, but at present I can only do about 10 minutes if I go every day.

Therapist: Well then, you will need to start at 10 minutes. Let's fill in the sections with the right amount of increase. It needs to be obvious what section you're in when you come to review your progress and then we can see how to set the onward levels (Table 6.2).

At his review the following week, Joshua had achieved getting information about art classes at his nearest centre but had not managed to

Table 6.2 Joshua's goal sheet

Score	Goal number 1 Art classes	Goal number 2 Daily walk
–2: least possible outcome	Do nothing	Less than 10 minutes daily
–1: what you can do now	Walk to library	10 minutes daily
0: expected level	Get leaflet about classes	11–14 minutes daily
+1: better than expected	Ring centres to get information	15–16 minutes daily
+2: best possible outcome	Get registered for a class	17 minutes or more daily
Score at review	+1	–1

Table 6.3 Joshua's second goal sheet, with a thought-challenging goal added

Score	Goal number 1 Art classes	Goal number 2 Daily walk	Goal number 3 Negative thoughts
–2: least possible outcome	Do nothing	Less than 10 minutes daily	Do nothing
–1: what you can do now	Read information about classes	13–14 minutes on two to six days a week; otherwise 10 minutes	Have negative thought, 'No one wants to meet me,' every day
0: expected level	Choose a class	13–14 minutes daily	Find evidence Invite a friend to my house
+1: better than expected	Ring centre to find out about registration	15–16 minutes on two to six days a week; otherwise 13–14 minutes	If successful invite two or more friends; if not, try a more likely friend
+2: best possible outcome	Get registered for a class	15–16 minutes daily	Have 'No one wants to meet me' thought less often than five times per week
Score at review			

increase his walking sufficiently. He had walked for 13 or 14 minutes on some days but not others.

Therapist: I think the walking goal needs to be re-scaled to allow for progress on two to six days per week. Possibly you could also review any negative thoughts that acted as barriers to your progress.

Joshua: I think I was held up by thinking no one would want to meet me at the pub.

Therapist: Let's add a thought-challenging goal. Now the form will look like this (Table 6.3).

Golden rule 4 – rewards

Keeping records is a very important part of pacing up your targets or you will soon get lost in your schedule and risk getting back on the roller coaster. Use the record form that Joshua filled in (he scored +1 for each goal at his next review, having found out which friends were available) or look at Jacky's further on in the chapter (see Table 6.4), or devise your own. Then reward yourself for having achieved your targets.

When you do think you have done well or even achieved just part of a target, congratulate yourself the same as you would your best friend. Possibly give yourself an extra treat. You might have achieved getting back to work for a few hours a week, or cooking a favourite meal for your partner who really appreciated your effort. So perhaps today is the day for buying the new shoes you saw last week but couldn't afford at the time.

Rewards are important to maintain motivation. Goals are best if they are rewarding in themselves, but if they involve chores or exercises that you know you 'should' do but cannot summon up the will for, use a technique called chaining.

Chaining works like this. You have been told to do exercises for upper body strengthening but you find them boring and uncomfortable. You want to achieve them to make progress but this is a longer-term reward and you need something that will help on a short-term, daily basis. Ask yourself what you most enjoy in the day: taking a bath, drinking coffee, watching a film on television, eating a meal with your family, doing meditation practice, or anything else that comes to mind. These activities are all rewards. (The technical term is reinforcers because they reinforce the activity that happens immediately before them.)

You can use this effect to make your exercises worthwhile. Do them immediately before your rewarding activity and tomorrow you will look forward to them instead of dreading the effort they take. The less preferred activity is 'chained' to a more preferred one and becomes associated with the pleasure in store.

Golden rule 5 – values

A new addition to the traditional behavioural component of CBT, which uses goal attainments in the ways we have discussed, concerns linking them to ongoing life values. Practitioners of acceptance and commitment therapy believe that goals need to be on their way to life-enhancing guiding principles. Values might involve improvement in self-care, intimate relationships, community activity, further education or care of others. The point of values is that they are never fulfilled because they imply a continuous commitment rather than completion of a specific task.

Table 6.4 Jacky's goal sheet

Value	Goal	Score	This week's targets	Thoughts that might stop me	Alternative thoughts
Self-improvement at work	Promotion	−2	Do nothing	She's too busy.	There is no
		−1	Email manager	I feel too anxious to ask	evidence that I won't
		0	Speak to manager	I don't suppose I'll succeed	succeed Jumping to
		+1	Speak to department head		conclusions is unhelpful I'll give it a
		+2	Arrange HR interview		try
Improvement in family relationships	Family outings	−2	Do nothing	There's the	Family outings are
		−1	Ask what they'd like	washing to do. I'll be too tired	important I'll risk
		0	Arrange zoo trip for Saturday, if agreed	We can't afford much money They might	feeling tired and disappointed if they don't
		+1	Zoo and restaurant lunch	not enjoy it after all	enjoy it It'll give me
		+2	Achieve Saturday trip and then go for a walk on Sunday as well		more information for next time

You might want to choose two or three goals from different value areas.

Jacky wanted to incorporate some of these ideas in recording her success with reaching her goals. She designed a form to note down how she was progressing towards her value-based goals of gaining a better job and spending more time with her family. She used the scoring system to gauge how much of the goal she had managed but included the reasons she might give herself for not reaching her expected outcome. This allowed her to identify the negative thoughts that might have prevented her progress and encouraged her to challenge them and keep focused on moving in the direction of her values (Table 6.4).

When Jacky met a friend who was also working on value based goals, in order to compare progress, she reported that she had managed to arrange an interview with her human resources manager and although her family hadn't done the Sunday walk they had gone to the zoo and had lunch there. She therefore gave herself a score of +2 for her first goal and +1 for the second – an overall achievement of +3 out of a total possible score of 4 and considerably better than her realistically expected score of 0. This increased her confidence at her promotion interview.

These are some ways in which you can change your life in spite of having a long-term disability. Choose really motivating goals, use a record form (see Table 6.1) and keep practising.

7

Communication and assertiveness

What is the purpose of communication? We need other people to understand us when we interact with them in a number of different ways. We are concerned with getting what we want or need and we like to maintain good social relationships. These are some of the functions of communication but they are not always successfully realized. It is often quite difficult to comprehend why people appear to misread our meaning and respond to us inappropriately.

Getting what you need

Disability brings a whole new dimension to what is already quite a tricky area. In the short term some people are anxious to help but gradually disappear. Others are embarrassed by the whole issue in case they say or do something wrong, and disappear instantly. Since you have acquired your disability you may consider that you have to carry a double responsibility – that of dealing with your own difficulties and at the same time trying to help others to feel at ease in your company.

The changed role that you might now find yourself playing in your social and family circle may involve altering your habitual style of interacting in order to show your friends and relatives how *they* can cope with the situation. This might be frustrating for you, especially if you find your efforts seem to make things worse.

Getting the help you need at the appropriate time is often a major concern, so trying to understand the viewpoint of your carers – those people who care for you and about you – is a good starting place. People attempt to convey their needs or opinions in different ways, which don't always get the response they intended. It might be a problem to do with their style of communication.

Communication styles

Try deciding which styles in the following list are more likely to be successful. Add any others which come to mind:

- Friendly
- Accusing
- Specific
- Non-judgemental
- Patient
- Apologetic
- Humorous
- Critical
- Listening
- Sympathetic.

In fact, as we shall see later, some of the styles that look as if they would be successful sometimes turn out to be irritating and alienating. Then we have to develop a whole new set of styles. I did warn you this was tricky!

Communicating with people you want something from

Anil, who had a serious back injury, wanted his family to appreciate his discomfort and make allowances for him when he had episodes of very bad pain. He used a number of strategies people often employ to communicate pain, but his wife Rena never quite seemed to respond as he wanted. He became increasingly irritable and the relationship

Table 7.1 Rena's reactions to Anil's behaviour, and Anil's responses

Anil's behaviour list	Rena's reaction	Anil's response
Sighing	Thinks she's done something wrong	Guilt, confusion
Rubbing	Feels irritated	Irritation
Grimacing	Rushes to help	Feel like a child, helpless
Withdrawing	Tries to interact with him, bring him out of it	Irritation, 'leave me alone'
Speaking sharply	Feels anxious and guilty	Have to reassure her
Staying in bed	Tries to motivate him	Guilt, anger
Complaining	Advises, tells him what to do	Disbelieved, incompetent
Frowning	Tries to cheer him up	Ignored, misunderstood

began to suffer. Eventually they went for couples CBT arranged by Anil's doctor, and they were both surprised by the results of an exercise that the therapist asked them to do. First, Anil was asked to list some of his pain communicating behaviours. Then, Rena was asked how she typically reacted to these. Finally, Anil had to disclose how he responded to her reactions. The therapist drew a grid (Table 7.1), and both Anil and his wife discovered how far off the mark their interaction had been.

Do you recognize any of the behaviours in Table 7.1? You can see from the chain of reactions that followed that Anil was unlikely to achieve what he wanted at the time. Besides, what he actually wanted is still a mystery – he hasn't yet told Rena how he wanted her to respond so she still feels helpless and tense. She could do with some specific information. Other people cannot know what you want unless you tell them accurately.

People who complain their partners should have known what to buy for a birthday present are liable to be disappointed, for people are not generally mind-readers. The information in Table 7.1 indicates how entangled interactions can become when needs and intentions are not clearly stated. Mind-reading is a form of cognitive distortion that we have met before in other chapters. In this example both partners made the same error. Anil's wife tried to read his mind and tried to respond according to what she thought he needed. Anil also tried mind-reading by assuming she knew what he wanted. The result was confusion and frustration.

Unfortunately patterns of communication like this can happen frequently and increase the problems involved in dealing with a disability. It can get even worse at times when distress is really high. At these times people tend to express themselves in really emotional ways and this can have the effect of being so overwhelming to others that they feel helpless in trying to deal with the situation and withdraw. At the very time you believe you are in need of the most support, people seem to be the least use.

Mary broke her pelvis in a serious fall and was never able to walk properly again. She had pins and plates in her bones and suffered a lot of discomfort as well as the frustration of needing to get about with crutches. She had previously been a successful salesperson but now the prospect of doing any kind of work seemed beyond her. Her mood was frequently low and even being sociable with her friends looked like too big an effort. After a few attempts at trying to involve her in their activities, her friends backed off because Mary had conveyed to them that she was too preoccupied with her disability to bother with them.

Mary then found herself being miserable and isolated as well as largely out of action. She often found herself thinking, 'Why can't they see that I need them to help me? All they do is rush away and have a good time without me.' What Mary really wanted was for her friends to visit her at home and help prepare a meal together, rather than take her out to places with difficult access. Because she thought they wouldn't want to visit her and because they had no idea that Mary would prefer a social meal at home, neither side achieved a solution.

Mary's problem was compounded by lack of assertiveness. Rather than risk having her friends reject her idea of eating at home, she would sometimes respond to their invitations to join them in a restaurant with answers like, 'I don't feel up to it and you will enjoy yourselves better without me. You go and have a good time.' At other times when she felt in a particularly low mood she would respond, 'You know I can't manage it. Why do you keep asking me? Just go and leave me alone,' which they did.

Mary became more miserable and angry with her friends for not helping her cope with her reduced ability. Eventually her friend Nicco, who was training as a therapist in CBT, saw the problem and decided to get Mary to state what would be best for her. He visited her one day determined not to be put off by her rejection. Their conversation went like this.

Nicco: Mary, I can see that going out for dinner is a problem for you. What would you prefer to do instead?

Mary: It's better if I stay home.

Nicco: Shall we all come and get a takeaway meal?

Mary: No, that's too expensive and not the sort of food I like.

Nicco: How do you normally get your shopping done so that you can have the food you like?

Mary: I get it delivered from the supermarket.

Nicco: That's a good idea. Would there be enough for a few of us to join you for dinner here?

Mary: Yes, but that's not what you would want to do. You all like going out. It's better if you leave me out of it.

Nicco: I think that's the problem, Mary. You don't really want to be left out but if you tell us to go without you, that's what we do. Then everyone feels miserable because we miss having you along.

Mary: Then that's your problem. Don't blame me if you don't have a good time.

Nicco (getting alongside Mary's mood): It's miserable for us all including you. We would like a better solution so we can all enjoy ourselves. We would like to eat here with you if that's easier for you. Would you like that too?

Mary: Yes, if you're sure, but I couldn't cook much of a meal.

Nicco: I think you could do with learning to tell people what you really want. We could have fun if you were to be head chef and we were your kitchen assistants! Then you could tell us how to prepare the dishes you have chosen.

Mary: I think that could work with a bit of practice. I could get some candles and it could be nicer than a posh restaurant in town.

And it was! So Nicco started the process of encouraging Mary to state her wishes directly by asking her to play a role so she wouldn't feel too awkward. This gave her a chance to practise the skills that she was going to need to get support for coping with her disability.

Let's look in more detail at the problems with Mary's previous communications. Sometimes she was too passive and at others too aggressive. Nicco wanted to show her that she needed to be assertive. These terms need defining.

- Passive: How do passive people ask for things? Usually by being too apologetic, speaking too quietly, showing submissive body postures and failing to get their point across. Mary's response of, 'You will enjoy yourselves better without me,' was too passive. She failed to get her needs met.
- Aggressive: How do aggressive people ask? Usually by being demanding and intimidating, showing their anger and failing to listen to the people they are interacting with. Mary's response, 'Why do you keep asking me? Go and leave me alone,' is an example. This also failed to meet her needs and alienated her friends' desire for her company as well.

Everyone deserves to be listened to – being assertive

The problem with both these approaches is that all the people in an interaction want their needs to be acknowledged. Passive people fail to get acknowledgement of their own needs. Aggressive people fail to acknowledge others' needs. Being assertive means stating your needs while respecting those of others.

So, if you want to be invited each time your friends go to dinner even if you sometimes need to refuse, it would be a bad idea to say either:

- 'You'd be best to go without me. I might spoil it for you' (this is too passive); or
- 'You never ask me to go with you. You're always rushing off without me' (this is too aggressive).

The assertive response might be: 'I really appreciate it when you invite me. Sometimes I can't get about so well, and I would prefer you to come here on those occasions, but I always like the opportunity to be included.' This makes clear that what you want is the option of choosing the venue. You have stated your need positively and respected their need to be 'kind' and want you to join in.

Sometimes people mistake passivity for 'being nice', wanting to make interactions smooth and pleasant and avoiding any chance of a confrontation. They already see themselves as a drain on their friends' time and attention so they are reluctant to suggest any solution that will seem to put their friends to any trouble. This runs the risk of a dangerous situation occurring where the behaviour suddenly flips from passive to aggressive.

Beware this passive–aggressive cycle. Frequently noticing that your needs are not being met will eventually lead to rebound aggressiveness.

Nicco understood this passive–aggressive cycle in Mary's behaviour and encouraged her to see that her angry response masked her despair at not keeping up with her friends. He was training in communication techniques so had an advantage over quite a few people you might find yourself interacting with.

If we return to Anil's example we find that his wife tried a number of roles in order to get the right response from him, but they produced rather the opposite effects.

The importance of personal responsibility

Anil needed to learn to convey to his wife, Rena, how he responded to her approaches and what he wanted instead. He also needed to respect her efforts to do the right thing, so the therapist advised him to set aside a time to discuss the problem with Rena. He was told to practise using 'I' statements to express his feelings directly and to take personal responsibility for them.

As we have frequently seen, when CBT strategies are used, the response to the situation depends on personal appraisal. If Anil had said, 'When you do that, you make me feel...,' he would have made Rena responsible for *his* evaluation of her effort. That seems rather unfair because her attempted behaviour followed from her judgement of what was needed. She wasn't given any direct information to help her do it any better. So Anil practised saying what he felt while getting alongside Rena's view of the situation, just as Nicco had done with Mary. He understood that Rena deserved to be listened to too.

So, if Rena rushed to assist he agreed to try saying, 'When it seems to me that you rush to help me, I know you are doing it for the best, but I feel rather like a child who needs things done for him. It would be best if you asked me first what to do and I'll try and tell you exactly what I need at that time.'

If Rena tried to motivate him to get out of bed he could say, 'I feel guilty lying in bed and I know it irritates you to think I'm just lazy, but if you try to get me up with promises of treats, I feel angry on top of everything else. I think it's best if you just leave me alone and go out with your friend. I'll feel better quicker if I have to make the effort to get my own meal!'

If Rena tried to advise him what to do he would tell her, 'When I think you are giving me advice, I know you are doing it to give me ideas, but I feel incompetent and I think you perhaps don't realize the effort I have already tried to make. It would be best if we could discuss what is most likely to be helpful on this occasion.'

If she seemed to be trying to entertain him he would say, 'I know that you are trying to cheer me up, but I feel rather as if you are trying to help me pretend I don't have a problem. I often feel anxious about my situation and I would prefer to practise relaxation instead.'

They discussed how his 'pain communication list' led to confusion and he agreed to ask Rena precisely for what he wanted her to do rather than hoping she would guess. If he didn't ask for anything, Rena agreed to do nothing and to leave him alone instead of trying to protect him from his discomfort.

Communicating with people who want something from you

A situation might arise in which you are asked to help someone else with a problem but your disability won't allow you to offer all the help they require. Remember, everyone wants to be listened to. Getting alongside their need helps to produce a workable solution.

Imagine this example. Your neighbour has to go to visit her elderly sick mother urgently. She asks you to walk her small son to school and fetch him home in the afternoon. You know you will not be able to do both journeys so you need to explain your situation to her. The passive response might be, 'I'm not well myself but I'll do my best.' This will fail to meet your own needs and runs the risk of making you resentful and possibly aggressive the next time. The aggressive response might be, 'You know I'm not well. Why do you always ask me to help you out?' This will fail to acknowledge her need and may alienate you from her friendship. She is less likely to be available if you need her to help you another time.

You need the three-point plan:

1 Acknowledge the other's need.
2 Acknowledge your need.
3 Negotiate a solution.

The assertive response might be:

- 'I can see you have a real problem today' (point 1).
- 'I don't think I can do both journeys' (point 2).
- 'If I do the morning walk, could you please ask Jane down the road to fetch your son home later?' (point 3).

This approach shows that you respect her needs in the situation as well as your own, and it will probably keep the neighbourhood relationships on a more sociable footing.

You can try the exercise that's about to follow but here are a few hints first:

- Stick to only one problem at a time.
- Ask friends or family members for an opportunity to discuss this problem.
- Agree that all solutions are on a trial basis to see how they work.

- When you want to point out how you feel in response to certain kinds of reactions, remember to use 'I' statements. 'You' statements sound accusing and others may feel defensive.
- Use statements such as: 'When...happens to me, I feel...,' (not, 'You make me feel...').
- Try to check your body posture (body language) to make it consistent with your statement – not too apologetic or aggressive. Look directly at the people you are addressing. Stand or sit facing them. Try to put your hands in an open gesture. If possible, avoid wrapping your arms round your body. This looks as if you are expecting to be treated like a victim. If you give people that cue, they may act on it!
- Try to be aware of unhelpful thoughts that prevent you acting assertively. Look out for thoughts such as, 'They should know how I feel,' or 'I don't deserve this.' Practise more permissive thoughts, such as, 'I would like them to do...and if they don't, it will not be the end of the world. I'll ask them what they would prefer and we can negotiate from there.'

Don't be afraid to practise. This strategy might not work out the first time but all behaviour experiments are 'no fail' – if you don't get success, what you do get is information that will help you try something different next time.

Here is an exercise you can try. Think of a situation in which you would like to communicate your needs assertively and avoid confrontation. Try to think of an easy problem to start with. Use this format as a guide to plan your approach:

- What is the problem you want to work on?
- How would you normally handle such a situation?
- How does it make you feel?
- What do you want to achieve?
- Work out what are your personal needs in the situation and what are the needs of others. (Remember the three-point plan here – acknowledge their need, acknowledge your need, negotiate a solution.)
- What would be the best assertive response?

Alex set himself the really difficult task of trying to get his parents to change their view that people with disabilities were inferior. He remembered overhearing adult conversations involving criticisms like this when he was a child and he was now dealing with his own disability as well as never having felt quite approved of by

Table 7.2 Alex's assertiveness exercise

Question	Response
What is the problem you want to work on?	I want to get my parents to stop thinking disabled people are inferior
How would you normally handle such a situation?	Tell them I think they are wrong but they won't agree with me
How does it make you feel?	Angry, rejected, unlovable, worthless
What do you want to achieve?	Get them to come to the gym and watch a few people in rehabilitation really working hard to achieve their goals
Work out what your personal needs are in the situation and what the needs of others are, using the three-point plan	
1 Acknowledge their need	They have held that view for a long time
2 Acknowledge your need	I need to feel approval from them
3 Negotiate a solution	Perhaps one visit to the gym won't be too hard for them
What would be the best assertive response?	I know you have the view that people with disabilities don't amount to much and I feel upset that you think the same of me. I probably used to think a bit the same but now I've experienced how much work rehabilitation takes, I've changed my mind. I would like it if you could see that too so I could believe you recognize the effort I'm making. Could you come to the gym on disability night so you can get firsthand knowledge?

his mother. He discussed this with his therapist and after several attempts he decided to 'get alongside' and acknowledge his parents' opinion before he could expect to modify it. His thinking is shown in Table 7.2.

Sally had a go at this exercise too. She wanted to go to an evening class but had trouble getting up the stairs to the classroom. She needed to get the college to recognize her problem and arrange a downstairs room instead. She filled in a form (Table 7.3) before going to the college authorities to remind her to be assertive rather than aggressive about the access arrangement.

As it turned out, the college authorities didn't move the class, but they informed Sally they were already aware of disability access and had installed a ramp and a lift at another entrance. Sally would have felt foolish if she had accused them of discrimination, but she did point out that the signposting was not very obvious. They agreed with this and added a better sign.

Table 7.3 Sally's assertiveness exercise

Question	Response
What is the problem you want to work on?	I want to have access to the language class
How would you normally handle such a situation?	Tell them I think they are guilty of disability discrimination if they don't change the room
How does it make you feel?	Angry, tense, ready for a fight, guilty that I need special treatment
What do you want to achieve?	I want to get the college people to put my class in a downstairs room for me
Work out what your personal needs are in the situation and what the needs of others are, using the three-point plan	
1 Acknowledge their need	They have already allocated the rooms and this will mess up their arrangements
2 Acknowledge your need	I need to get into the class
3 Negotiate a solution	Perhaps they wouldn't mind swapping with one other class
What would be the best assertive response?	Thank you for seeing me. I need to ask if there is a way I could get to the Thursday night language class. I feel excluded because I can't manage stairs. I know you have already allocated the rooms but I would really like to join that class. Is there some way it could move to a ground floor room?

You can have a go at filling in a form like Alex's and Sally's if you have a problem like theirs that needs solving. Maybe, for example, you need to get more help from your local council, medical practice or litigation team if you are applying for compensation after your injury.

See if you can identify how other people act assertively. Can you learn anything from their style? Often using someone else as your model will help you to 'play the role' initially until you find your own style to fit.

8

Stress and its effects on managing long-term disability

What is the stress response? It is a three-part reaction to an event or situation that *you think* you can't cope with. It can be expressed as the demands of a situation divided by your perceived resources to deal with it. If you believe your resources are insufficient to meet the demands of a stressor such as manoeuvring your wheelchair in an unfamiliar enclosed space, you will feel the symptoms of stress when confronted with that situation.

The three parts to the stress response are:

- cognitive – thoughts, beliefs and images about the situation and your own abilities;
- biological – increased heart rate, muscle tension, stress hormones, lowered immune system;
- emotional – anxiety, sadness, anger, depression, shame.

Where do you feel it? Many body systems are involved.

These reactions are all intended to make the body ready for action to deal with attack. Adrenal glands in the back of the abdomen, directed by the pituitary gland in the brain, produce adrenalin and cortisol. These prepare the body to accelerate and fight or run away. This response was appropriate in the past, when the early part of the human brain was developing thousands of years ago. People, like animals, had to be able to deal successfully with all kinds of challenges in order to survive and pass on their genes. The heart rate speeds up to send more blood to the muscles. Breathing increases to boost the amount of oxygen available. Digestion stops, since it is less important. This causes discomfort in the stomach and the need to empty bowels and bladder to make the body lighter. The brain may have lots of thoughts rushing about, which may help to form a solution. Sweating allows the body to cool.

These effects can make a person capable of activities using intense amounts of energy but they need to be short-lived, and the body needs to rest afterwards. The problem arises when the situation is not resolved by using the high levels of energy these reactions produce and the body remains in an extremely alert, stressed state. The biological changes then become long term (chronic) and the effects may become harmful rather than useful. The rushing thoughts lead to confusion and headache. Increased breathing rates lead to an imbalance of the normal gases in the blood and cause dizziness and a sense of breathlessness. This can also result in numbness and tingling around the mouth and in the ends of the fingers. The digestive changes can become long-lasting, leading to decreased appetite and weight loss, though sometimes people respond to these sensations by eating more and then gaining excessive weight. Muscles that are poised ready for action but are not exercised can become stiff, tense and painful.

What causes stress? People report many situations in modern life that make them feel stressed and anxious. Among these are relationship problems, illness, injury, change, pain, overwork, noise and boredom. From the point of view of coping with a disability, you may experience most of these at the same time and you may begin to think you will never achieve a more settled lifestyle.

Maria experienced these sensations when she considered going out alone and started to have panic attacks. You will remember that she imagined she would fall out of her wheelchair and no one would help her. She also thought she might have a heart attack. By identifying the distortions in her thinking and carrying out a behavioural experiment she was able to learn that the situation did not demand more resources than she already had, and her stress response reduced.

So, the way you interpret situations may signal that a stressor exists and prepare the body for fight or flight. You may then have strategies that have proved to be useful in the past so the stress response reduces. If this is not the case, the condition may get worse with each stressor (Figure 8.1).

The fight or flight is not really appropriate for a stressor such as manoeuvring your wheelchair. The brain has interpreted the situation as beyond your resources and has set the reaction off by mistake. As well as noticing your pounding heart and exhausted muscles in situations like this, you may also find over time that the stress response affects your immune system, so you may be likely to get more illnesses if you are in a state of constant stress. The body may attempt to return to normal but the levels of the hormones remain high if your attempts at coping are not effective.

The symptoms of stress are not very pleasant if they occur when you need to think calmly about a problem like doing the shopping. People will tend to avoid the situation that sets the alarm reaction off and any situations like it, becoming more limited in the activities they actually

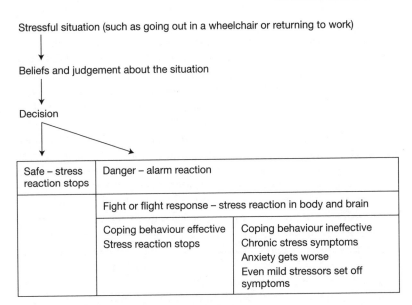

Figure 8.1 shows a flowchart:

Stressful situation (such as going out in a wheelchair or returning to work)
↓
Beliefs and judgement about the situation
↓
Decision
↓

Safe – stress reaction stops	Danger – alarm reaction	
	Fight or flight response – stress reaction in body and brain	
	Coping behaviour effective Stress reaction stops	Coping behaviour ineffective Chronic stress symptoms Anxiety gets worse Even mild stressors set off symptoms

Figure 8.1 Responses to stressful situations

do. This is quite a frequent state of affairs and will happen readily in response to a panic attack once it has been experienced. Shopping is the most common example, with the supermarket the most likely place for the panic attack to occur. After this, people will avoid the supermarket and may gradually avoid all kinds of shops or crowded places. Actually, this is the true meaning of agoraphobia – fear of the market place.

This is called 'fear avoidance' and gets in the way of lots of goals that may be important.

Josef had an accident at work when a forklift truck ran over his foot, crushing it badly and damaging the bones and blood vessels in his lower leg. He had a below-knee (transtibial) amputation. Mostly he has coped well with his disability but he gets anxious about walking around his local shopping centre in the way that he used to be able to do. On one occasion he walked too far and felt panicky about being able to get home safely. He went to his doctor who told him to rest until he felt better. The next time Josef tried to walk he was out of condition and could go less far before he began to notice his heart pounding and felt breathless. He became fearful that his situation had deteriorated and he walked less and less until eventually he couldn't leave the house without having a lot of stress symptoms. He learned to be afraid of the activity he used to enjoy, and he needed advice.

Josef's response was probably based on the cognitive distortions we have met before. Unfortunately some people compound their problems by responding to their stressors with self-medication of one sort or another and so can sometimes end up with addiction as well. That is often the case if PTSD goes untreated for a long time. As we saw in Omar's case, high levels of anxiety and distress are common after a life-threatening event. The situation was even worse for Kieran.

Kieran was a serving soldier in the army with many years' experience of combat in various theatres of war over the time of his career. He was naturally exposed to scenes of horrific injuries in both civilians and members of his own unit. He was wounded himself but after medical treatment and rehabilitation at military medical establishments, he was considered fit to return to duty on each occasion. He was aware of feeling depressed but thought little of it as high morale is essential in motivating his colleagues and he believed that complaining would be considered a sign of cowardice. He continued with his duties for eight years but tried out various drugs whenever he could, and he found that they sometimes helped him to deal with his mood problems and the need to be constantly vigilant about the safety of his unit. He also found that alcohol helped him initially, but gradually he started to drink so much that his colleagues were worried about him. He became violent and unpredictable on occasions and he was eventually discharged from the army for disciplinary reasons.

He returned to live with his wife but his situation continued to deteriorate and she encouraged him to see his doctor. Unfortunately this doctor was unclear about his problem and only offered him antidepressant medication, which did little to help. Because Kieran was now using quite high doses of illegal drugs, he soon came to the attention of the police and found himself in court. His family was horrified and could not understand how a well-respected soldier who had been decorated for bravery in two combat operations and had suffered injuries in the pursuit of protecting his country was now being treated as a criminal.

At this point, Kieran was referred for psychiatric reports because the magistrates were aware of media articles about PTSD in service personnel. This was diagnosed and Kieran was placed on a waiting list for CBT, but he had to wait until National Health Service (NHS) resources were available. This delay compounded the problem and Kieran lost hope of ever recovering. He committed suicide.

As a result of this, his family tried to raise the awareness of the Ministry of Defence to the plight of serving soldiers who have been subjected to multiple traumas. Gradually, the condition has come to be more readily recognized and more facilities are being made available.

Table 8.1 Some good and bad responses to stress

Response	Good	Bad
Drugs (such as tranquillizers, painkillers)		✓
Alcohol		✓
Smoking		✓
Caffeine drinks		✓
Exercise	✓	
Relaxation	✓	
Self-talk, reinterpretation	✓	

Military medical units are now equipped to assess wounded service personnel for psychological as well as physical injury, and treatment programmes are now being set up in collaboration with NHS mental health staff. Kieran's family believe they have at least helped to bring this about and have spoken to Kieran's colleagues in his army unit to make sure that they seek appropriate help at a much earlier stage.

If you think you might be at risk of PTSD, go to your doctor as soon as you can and refer to the list of further resources at the end of this book if necessary.

You can see from this example that some responses to stress are worse than others. There are some things you can do which are more effective (Table 8.1).

Exercise is useful because it burns up the energy stored in the muscles, including the heart, and can increase a sense of well-being, which will allow you to view the stressor in a more positive light. Learning a system of relaxation is also a good idea. You might have discovered this already from your rehabilitation therapists or you might like to look ahead to Chapter 9 (on mindfulness and meditation) and Chapter 12 (on treatments for phantom sensations, which include scripts for deep relaxation exercises). These help the physiological symptoms as well as the emotional ones. Looking at some of the ways you can explore your interpretation of the situation to see if you can challenge your more negative beliefs will enable you to change your self-talk so that it is more likely to encourage you to cope. Like Maria, Josef found out about the stress response and the ways to challenge anxiety-producing thoughts. He filled in a record form like the one in Table 8.2.

He learned that it's important to help the brain to interpret the situation more realistically. His heart rate increased partly because he was expending energy and so needed more oxygen for his walk but also because, as he later recognized, the symptoms were due to anxiety rather than an impending heart attack. Once he was convinced of this

Table 8.2 Josef's thoughts and emotions when walking around the shopping centre, and alternative thoughts and responses

Thoughts	Emotion	Alternative thoughts	Response
My heart's beating so fast I'm sure I'll have a heart attack	Anxiety, panic	My heart's racing because I assume I'm in danger. It is preparing me for 'fight or flight', but I don't need that here	I'll sit down, practise breathing calmly and wait for the feelings to pass

Then I will go home when I feel ready

I have always succeeded at shopping in the past so I have no evidence to assume a disaster will occur |

he was able to practise the relaxation techniques he had learned and continue with his shopping trip more comfortably.

Think of a stressful event yourself. Remember many stressors exist that are not necessarily a result of your disability but are now more difficult to cope with – for example, family events like weddings or religious festivals. How would you normally deal with such a situation? Which of the responses in Table 8.1 are you most likely to use? How would you rate your thoughts about it? Can you think of more helpful beliefs? Practise trying to avoid responses that increase the stress response. In particular, look for self-talk that reminds you how you have coped successfully in the past. Consider the situation, your thoughts, your emotions, your alternative thoughts, and your response, as in Josef's form.

9

Mindfulness-based CBT

The new CBT is ACT

What is ACT? This stands for acceptance and commitment therapy, which has its focus on giving up the struggle to achieve some other state and instead to experience how things are at this moment in an accepting, non-judgemental fashion. It is not the same as resigning yourself to assuming the situation cannot change, nor is it just giving up any attempt to improve things. It is an active process involving committing yourself to accept some emotional pain (since just being alive makes us vulnerable to this) and living with how things change moment to moment rather than trying to force things to be as we would like them to be.

How is ACT different from what we used to know?

Throughout this book we have been dealing with the influence of thoughts on feelings and actions. In Chapter 4 we looked at the persistent quality of intrusive thoughts in post-traumatic stress disorder and discovered that thought suppression (trying to un-think thoughts or distract yourself from them) is not effective. Unhelpful thoughts and beliefs will constantly reappear and are an important focus of therapy in both CBT and ACT. Traditional cognitive therapy techniques deal with how we think about things and interpret events. Therapists ask people to find meaning in the thoughts, encourage evaluation, focus on evidence and reinforce the notion that thoughts and feelings lead to actions. ACT prefers to consider how we experience the thoughts themselves, to encourage us to learn that thoughts have a behaviour of their own. ACT also seeks to undermine the power of language. As we shall see later, words carry meanings that spread beyond the current moment-to-moment experience.

One of the ways CBT can work is by changing the content of thoughts. ACT believes that it could also be possible to change people's response to negative thoughts and feelings. Identifying negative thoughts as they arise and standing back to examine their content can allow people to shift their perspective on the thoughts. Instead of being regarded as true, thoughts and feelings can be experienced as passing events in the mind – neither necessarily a true reflection of reality nor central aspects of the self. People who have tried it often report that this gives them an enormous sense of relief.

Both CBT and ACT use behavioural activities as a means of helping people move towards their preferred goals. As we saw in Chapter 6, goals may be specific behaviours on their way to life-enhancing principles. ACT sessions ask participants if they believe they are moving in a value direction rather than just achieving particular goals.

However, the basic techniques of ACT have more to do with 'mindfulness' and meditation than has previously been the case with CBT. It emphasizes the importance of remaining in the present and resisting the old habits of the downward spiral of thoughts and emotions.

Mindfulness has come to us from Buddhist meditative practice and is now gaining universal appeal. Its main purpose is to do with improving our capacity for paying attention and gaining a new perspective on the things that drive us. It is a way of *being* rather than *doing*. It teaches us self-observation, allowing us to suspend the habit of characterizing, evaluating and judging ourselves with our old familiar automatic thought processes and emotional reactions.

Rumination about the negative aspects of a problem for which there is no ready solution can take over much of our thinking space. The mind continues to process the problem in 'doing' mode and becomes so busy with the past and future that it becomes unaware of the present.

In Chapter 8 I discussed the effects of stress on managing long-term disability. Maybe you are still stressed by thoughts about failure and worthlessness from time to time. Trying to 'fix' these problems risks you getting sucked back into old habits of matching yourself with some ideal standard and falling short. There are no standards, as we discovered when we looked at problems with self-esteem in Chapter 5.

Omar, who suffered post-traumatic stress disorder, worked hard at confronting the intrusive memories, and no longer avoids situations that remind him of his injury. Nevertheless he still sometimes finds himself asking the 'why me?' question. Although he knows there is no answer, his thoughts tend in that direction when his mood is low because of a setback during the day. Omar decided to learn some mindfulness techniques in order to 'let go' of the question, rather than trying to formulate an answer. He learned that in 'being' mode the mind has nothing to do except directly experience the present.

Breath of life

For centuries people have used breathing as a vehicle for meditation. Mindfulness meditation aims to increase awareness of present moment-to-moment experience, bringing attention back to the present using focus on the breath as an anchor whenever the attention wanders.

Classes in mindfulness meditation usually contain an exercise called 'body scan'. Exercises like this were developed as the basis of a stress management programme for people with all kinds of physical illnesses and disabilities. The programme was created by Dr Jon Kabat-Zinn in Massachusetts and it has been considered so effective that its influence has spread to other countries and is used by therapists working with sufferers of mental as well as physical illness and pain problems. You can try the meditation exercise below as an example, but official programmes request that you follow the technique with a tape and practise for 45 minutes every day. This is why a central part of ACT is commitment! However, Dr Kabat-Zinn has found that once people get into it they continue to use meditation daily for many years.

Body scan is used to bring awareness of sensations throughout the whole body, using the breath as a vehicle to carry awareness into regions of the body where the sensations may have greater intensity – breathing into them.

Body scan meditation

Important note: do not practise this while driving or attempting any task that requires your attention.

1 Take up a comfortable position, sitting on a chair or lying down.
2 Focus on movements of your breath in and out of your body.
3 Notice where your body touches the chair (or bed or floor).
4 Bring awareness to your lower abdomen as you breathe in and out.
5 Feel or imagine your breath entering the abdomen and all down your legs. On the out breath, feel the breath coming all the way back.
6 Bring awareness to each part of the body in turn by feeling or imagining the breath entering those body areas. See if there are any sensations in any particular body regions. Just notice them. If there are no sensations, just notice that.
7 If you become aware of tension in any muscle group, focus attention specifically on it, following the breath into those particular muscle groups. 'Breathe in' to those areas and release the tension on the out breath.

8 The mind will wander (minds like to be busy). Each time you notice, guide your mind back to the last body part you remember being aware of and pick the scan up again in the next moment, with the next breath, as often as necessary.

Focusing on the breath brings you back to living in this present moment instead of reliving the past ('I was a fool to have done that') or pre-living the future ('It will always be the same'). Breath is always available to be of use to you. No special place or equipment, no expensive subscriptions to a fitness centre are required. Breath is truly the miracle of life.

As you become more experienced you can extend the meditation to become aware of your thoughts. Negative thoughts and feelings are often expressed through the body as stress responses. Breathing can be used to settle physical responses so that the thoughts can be examined calmly.

Thoughts are not facts. You can experience them like you experience the sensations of the chair you are sitting on against your body. The chair is not part of you. The thoughts are not you. You can choose to let them pass through and change, just as the sensations of your body against the chair change over the time you are sitting.

When you are ready, bring your attention away from your body sensations to your thought stream, noticing how thoughts arise and pass through your mind space. Notice their quality but escort your mind away from attaching meaning to them and bring it back to observation of the thoughts. Become aware of automatic thoughts without judging them so as not to be carried away with them. You may want to follow where your thoughts have taken you. Facing what is present and acknowledging difficulties is the most effective way of reducing rumination about how you would prefer things to be. Let go of this struggle and see if you can allow yourself to feel what you feel. Notice all the sensations in the body; notice each one and let it pass along. Notice emotions and thoughts; notice each one and let it pass along.

The witness and the stream

If you can do this rather difficult and challenging exercise, you will have noticed that there is a part of yourself that is observing and labelling the thinking. This is you as your witness. You are observing the thoughts but are untouched by their content. The witness is the stable core that observes the passing stream of thought and emotion.

An example that is commonly used in mindfulness exercises is that of the witness as a bus, with you as both the bus and the driver. You are driving the bus in the direction of your valued goals but the bus is full of 'thought passengers' who keep reminding you of the habitual judgements you make about yourself and your future: 'It'll never work,' 'I'm not good enough,' and other such ideas that may have driven you off course before. The bus contains the passengers in the same way that you contain the thoughts, but the thoughts are not 'you' in the same way that the bus is not the passengers. You can witness the passengers and choose to let them off the bus while you continue in your preferred direction.

Cognitive defusion

In earlier chapters we explored the way in which interpretation of events appear to be glued or fused to their related emotional and behavioural consequences. ACT encourages us to undo or 'defuse' this process by recognizing that thoughts are just passing mind events that don't in themselves carry any power to cause a reaction.

Previously you may have reacted to a thought with self-judgements, which also come along on the thought stream. ('This is no good. I can't concentrate.' 'I'm a failure at this. I'll never get any good at it.') This demonstrates the old habit of getting caught up in the thoughts. The thought ('I can't concentrate') has become entangled with the judgement process, which has moved it along from a passing event in the mind to a core belief in personal failure and hopelessness for the future. The mind has wandered down its old familiar path and may have caused the mood to change in sympathy. Therefore it is important to explore what's going on in this stream of associations so as to disengage the thought from the judgement.

Stop, step back, refocus on your breath. The breath always gives a chance to begin again. It is always available for a new beginning, always new in this moment. Notice the thought. ('There's that thought again.') There is no need to fix anything because thoughts do not represent the whole truth about you. Instead of jumping in to try and solve the problem, stand back to see what it feels like to see the problem without reacting. Use your breath to find a calm place from which to observe it. Just notice and see if by separating the thought, 'I can't concentrate,' from the judgement, 'I am a failure,' the stream of thoughts will pass by without sucking you into the old process of emotional reaction and behavioural response. Acknowledge the judgement for what it is – a mental event, just a thing in the mind, not something imposed from outside. Just watch the mind as it moves and take an accepting, non-judgemental approach to what you notice. Notice the stream passing along. If it disappears, you are caught up in the content of the thought and are processing rather than observing, doing rather than being. Try to refocus attention by coming back again and again to the breath. The core skill is to acknowledge and step out of the old spirals of thoughts, emotions, moods and self-perpetuating responses.

Thoughts might also be like clouds passing across the sky. They pass through and change without changing the sky itself. If you stop and think about a cloud you can choose options about how to react rather than assuming that a deluge is imminent and it will all end in disaster.

There is normally a choice of actions you can take if you examine thoughts as if they were passing clouds. Does it look like rain? Shall I react by taking an umbrella or take a chance of getting wet? In Jacky's case (see Chapter 6), she decided to choose going to the zoo and coping with feeling tired and disappointed rather than avoiding the opportunity of a family outing.

The speeding car experiment

Now you have had a chance to experience what mindfulness and meditation are trying to achieve, look again at the power of words. Practise the body scan again (see pp. 77–8). Pay attention to the rate of your breathing – keep it slow and natural. Also notice your heart beat. This will also be slow and comfortable as you keep your attention on your breath.

Now imagine a car driving down your street at top speed. It is going so fast it will crash into people on the pavement. Allow your mind to focus on the speeding car.

What has happened to your breathing and your heart rate? Turn your attention back to them. You will probably notice they have speeded up too. Now open your eyes and refocus on the room you are in. There is no car and no injured people. The reactions in your body responded to the words 'speeding car' in your mind. The words carried almost the same reactions as the actual event and conjured it up. You could label the feelings as anxiety. Anxiety says something is dangerous but it's just a word describing thoughts and feelings. In this case it was a word to describe a reaction to other words. Thoughts often contain words and these can come to represent the whole of a situation. These thoughts may have been learned from your early experiences, as Joshua found in Chapter 2. They can allow you to conjure up your early experiences of a critical person and you can be carried along with them. They can spread out so that childhood experiences reappear in adulthood, but they don't represent the whole identity of the person, the whole reality as it applies to this current moment. New experiences have shaped the self along the way. This is not reality. Thoughts are not facts. Words are not our masters.

Look at barriers to achieving progress toward values. Notice the barriers are just words – anxiety, exhaustion and so on. You can have these but still carry out valued behaviours.

You can choose to take your family to the zoo (consistent with value) and choose to endure any stress associated with the outing. We can't always choose how we feel but we can choose our willingness to experience it like Jacky decided to do.

If thoughts are chaotic, BREATHE: take a Breathing space, Refocus on the breath, Experience and Attend to the Thoughts, Hold the sensations in the mind space produced by the breath, and Escort your mind back as often as necessary. Allow thoughts to progress across your mind rather than getting them stuck in a spiral. There is a possibility that just noticing this process might reduce the chaos and lead to a solution. Whatever happens observe and accept it, acknowledging judgement thoughts to be just a part of the procession.

Once you're very practised at this you can use a breathing space many times a day, whenever you feel overwhelmed or notice your mood lowering or your usual triggers for negative ruminations about your disability.

Remind yourself of these steps:

Break off from current activity or thought.
Refocus attention on the breath.
Experience whatever is happening in the body mindfully.
Attend to the sensations without judging them.
Think the thoughts that come up as mental events that are passing through.
Hold all the sensations in the space created by the breath.
Escort the mind back as often as necessary to the breath.

10

Personal relationships and sex in long-term disability

No sex please, we have a disability, and other myths

- You can't be sexy if you're disabled.
- If you need help because of your disability, you are a child and too immature to have a sex life.
- Disabled people need protection.
- Real sex involves penetration.
- Penises are always erect and ready.
- Both partners should have simultaneous orgasms every time.
- People who want sex with a disabled person are perverts.
- Masturbation is wrong.
- Men can always tell when women reach orgasm.
- If there are sexual problems in a relationship with a disabled person, they are always the result of the disability.

In a relationship in which there is trust and honesty, intimacy is the process by which people exchange feelings, thoughts and actions. This doesn't need to imply sexual intercourse or even a sexual encounter at all. Workshops on intimacy and relationships sometimes ask participants to do a homework assignment in which they must ask a close member of their family, 'What specific thing must I do to show you I love you?'

You might think hugs and kisses are top choices but here are some recent actual responses:

- Water my garden for me (from a young daughter).
- Take me shopping with you (from a teenage son).
- Watch this film with me (from a husband).
- Offer to make me a cup of tea when I get home later than you (from a wife).

These would not be your immediate expectations of highest priority behaviours, but they reveal individual preferences and the extremely misleading error of mind-reading, which we have met before. Sex is just one component of personal relationships but it seems to be particularly exposed to other people's assumptions about individual interactions, especially if one or both partners have a disability.

Rehabilitation programmes don't always include sufficient attention to ongoing sexual needs. Perhaps staff attitudes and training are too restricted. Sex is an important part of a good quality of life and while disability may mean ways of expression may change, it remains an activity of daily living, like doing the washing from a wheelchair or the shopping from a mobility scooter – the methods have been adjusted to provide a solution to the problem.

Each culture will determine what is acceptable according to its moral and religious traditions. These change not only in place but also in time so that each generation in the 'Western' world may seem more sexually open and experimental than the preceding one. While some believe that this is leading to disaster, and that AIDS is the current price to be paid, repressive views of sexual behaviour can be damaging to people's true human development and are in contrast to historical perspectives of vitality, particularly those from earlier cultures. People have a right to sexual experience and privacy to develop their fullest potential, to choose their partner status and to make their own decisions. Every person has sexual feelings, attitudes and beliefs. Sex is a natural function controlled largely by reflexive responses of the body so the focus needs to be on minimizing any blocks to effective expression.

Other factors besides the disability itself may reduce the possibility of good sexual communication, so problems such as anger or self-esteem issues might have to take priority before any sexual difficulty can be successfully addressed. Where mood problems are a significant part of any sexual dysfunction, they should be treated as a main concern, in the ways that we have been considering.

The importance of good self-esteem

Media representations of sexuality show a fantasy idea of athleticism and attraction and of being in a continuous state of readiness, so anxieties about personal attractiveness can be heightened by everyday exposure to television and magazine articles. This is bad enough for those of us who just get older without the added difficulty of acquiring a disability along the way. Where adjustment to a disability also includes experiences of anger and anxiety, sexual performance can be further reduced. In addition, psychological problems may predate the onset of disability because of restricted upbringing practices or sexual abuse in earlier life. As a result of performance anxiety, you may then become so preoccupied with signs of your own or your partner's arousal that you become less and less involved in the interaction itself. The pattern of reactions may start to look like the depiction in Figure 10.1.

The anxiety might generalize to all potential situations where sex could occur and lead to consequences such as avoidance of any affectionate behaviour, or engagement in only transient liaisons so as to

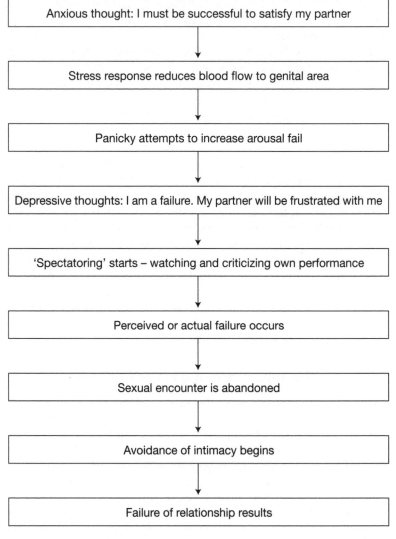

Figure 10.1 Possible spiral of events in sexual performance anxiety

avoid the demands of a relationship. People who fear rejection sometimes evade intimacy, preferring superficial relationships that avoid the
risks of commitment. Acquiring a disability may make this perception
even more acute.

Sally had a number of unsuccessful relationships before her amputation and dreaded the reaction of her current partner after her accident.
She hated the appearance of her residual limb (stump) and actually had
more negative feelings about it than her partner. The scarring made
her self-conscious about her appearance in general and significantly
reduced her vulnerable self-esteem. Initially she kept her affected leg
hidden whenever her partner tried to engage in a romantic encounter
and she tried to discourage it. Gradually, however, as her partner
seemed to insist on including this leg when giving her a massage, Sally
became more confident about accepting her changed body and learned
to admire the neatness of the surgical scars and the ability of her small
limb to control her artificial leg and walk short distances. She learned
to be more trusting in the relationship and more experimental in
giving and receiving affection.

So, sexual health needs to integrate psychological and emotional
dimensions as well as physical ones, but there are considerable changes
to be addressed in certain kinds of disability, particularly if it is associated with neurological damage to the central nervous system (brain
and spinal cord). The spinal cord transmits physical sensations to the
brain and participates in all reflexes. The impact of any neurological
damage depends on the level of injury. Brain injuries can affect sexual
expression, reduce normal inhibition and cause changes in memory
and mood. Injury to the lower brain areas including the hypothalamus
may result in hormone changes. The hormones testosterone and oes-
trogen both occur in both sexes and hormonal problems can affect
sexual appetite and performance in ways that are similar in both men
and women.

Diabetes and vascular illness will also cause erectile and lubrication
problems, though not necessarily reduction of appetite or ejaculation.

Drugs such as antihypertensives, antidepressants, opiates, some
tranquillizers and high or even moderate doses of alcohol reduce sexual
appetite and pleasure.

Spinal cord injury will lead to changes in sexual response, depending
on the completeness of the injury and what areas of the spinal cord are
affected. Complete spinal cord injury will cause loss of erections in men
and loss of lubrication in women in response to arousing fantasies,
sounds or sights. Most people with spinal cord injury will experience
reflex erections or lubrication in response to direct touch but they

will be unaware of this as they have no sensation below the level of the injury and these reflexes are usually not useful in the context of a sexual encounter. Men with incomplete lesions can often achieve a partial erection which may be sufficient for intercourse with a helpful partner.

Women with complete spinal cord injury will generally recover normal fertility and can become pregnant but will lose sensation and lubrication in the genital area. Women can still have intercourse and may actively encourage it to retain a sense of normality but must be aware of any sense of being exploited or treated as sexually passive.

Vibrators and other sex toys are useful in exploring sexually sensitive areas of the body, though women rarely like to introduce objects into their vaginas even if they have sensation. Surveys show that most women prefer stimulation around the outside of the clitoral area rather than insertion into the vagina, and they need to convey this to their partner who might believe penetration is the only true way to help them to orgasm.

Erectile dysfunction may be treatable with injections or devices to prevent blood flowing back out of the penis. In women, dryness can be overcome with lubricants such as surgical jelly or saliva if that appeals to you both. Erections and lubrication are not all there is to sex, however. Both spinal-cord-injured men and women can experience orgasm, though ejaculation is significantly affected (possibly in both sexes according to recent research). Ejaculation and orgasm are separate things. Orgasm is a sense of release associated with muscle contractions, which can occur in response to cuddling, kissing and massaging unaffected parts of the body.

Leroy, who has a spinal injury from a mountaineering accident and is now paralysed, has no sensation from above the waist downwards. He has had extensive rehabilitation and manages his bowel, bladder and pressure area problems successfully. He is exploring his changed sexual responses as he cannot feel if his partner is touching him in his affected areas. In fact, he has most response from erotic touch around his neck and upper chest. Along with verbal and visual stimulation from his partner and sometimes the use of a vibrator he can experience orgasm, and with close body contact he can also satisfy his partner.

Polio, being a condition that affects muscles rather than nerves, may reduce the ability to move but not sensation.

Ella has a different kind of paralysis from Leroy's. She had polio as a child and her muscles grew weaker as she got older (the post-polio syndrome). She cannot now move her lower body. However, as sensation is not affected she can have orgasm during intercourse if she chooses by using supportive pillows to get herself into the most comfortable position. She likes to keep eye contact with her partner and often chooses a side-to-side position.

Pain reduces the appetite for sex and the choice of positions in both sexes. This can lead to avoidance of sexual activity but, on the other hand, rewarding activity is a major pain management strategy, as we saw in Chapter 6. You may need to experiment with positions, stimulators and timing. Learning to focus on the moment, as in 'mindfulness', or on a sexual fantasy can distract you from the pain and allow you to concentrate on your reactions and those of your partner.

The importance of good communication

Choosing partners may be more than usually important if you believe there is a risk of exploitation. As you would normally, check out the track record of a potential partner's relationships and how they ended. What do their friends say about people you regard as potential partners? Have they only ever dated people with disabilities? Are they devotees (people who need the fantasy or reality of a disabled partner to gain arousal)? Is that OK with you? If you're fairly satisfied that a particular person is interesting, don't be afraid to make the first move. You may have to take responsibility for undoing non-disabled people's prejudices and to let them see that you have normal needs for affection and intimacy.

People in relationships often don't have all the information they need and will fill in the blanks with their own beliefs, but good communication will allow for choices to be discussed, can be a part of comfortable intimacy and will relieve the partner of the need to guess (or mind-read!).

Men's arousal is visible by the degree of erection while women's is less obvious. In a heterosexual interaction a woman may believe the erection has to be 'looked after' and might indicate acceptance of penetration. The man can only *assume* she is sufficiently ready and therefore she must take responsibility for signalling her own needs. A man with a female partner often has no idea where the woman 'is'. She may assume he knows and then feel angry that he doesn't show consideration – although she has already given him the signal to proceed. She may fear that if she asks him to delay while she becomes more aroused he may reject her in favour of someone more compliant. She might believe he feels threatened if he's expected to maintain his erection while she takes longer to get aroused. It seems that some assertive communication could be helpful, and you might want to review Chapter 7.

If you like to use a vibrator and you want to incorporate it into sexual activity with your partner, make sure you both agree so that your partner doesn't assume that you intend giving a 'you're inadequate' message.

Use language stating, 'I would prefer...' as much as possible to avoid seeming to blame your partner for your lack of response. Non-verbal messages may also be particularly useful in sexual interaction to show what you prefer. For example, take your partner's hand and guide it to show what's especially stimulating at any given time. Using this technique (called hand riding) to pace arousal by encouraging stopping and starting may enhance pleasure for both of you.

Exploring your own changed responses

It is a good idea to use masturbation to discover which parts of your body are now sensitive to erotic touch. Use vibrators if necessary and don't forget the power of imagination – remember the speeding car experiment in Chapter 9 – your body (though not necessarily your genital area) will respond just to the idea.

Pat and Sam, who both have pain and movement problems following injury in a road accident, decided to try a technique called sensate focus. This was first described by Drs Masters and Johnson in the 1970s but soon became widespread. It is a set of steps towards the most effective form of sexual communication for each partner, starting from a very relaxed situation in which there is no demand to succeed so there is no threat of failure. It allows you to build up knowledge of what pleases you and your partner without anxiety, guesswork or 'spectatoring' – watching and criticizing your performance. Let's see how they did it. You can choose to assign a sex to each partner depending on your own preferences.

Pat lies face down, using pillows for support. Sam strokes Pat's back starting from the neck and working down to Pat's feet, concentrating on what it feels like to touch Pat's skin. Pat focuses attention on the sensations as Sam does the caressing. Pat tells Sam what feels good and whether the caress is too fast, heavy, slow or light. Pat does not have to worry about whether Sam is getting tired, aroused or bored, it is the receiving partner's responsibility just to experience the touch and notice which areas of the body are particularly responsive.

When Pat turns over, Sam can continue stroking but this time down the front of the body. At this stage it is important to avoid directly touching the genital areas.

When they are both ready, they change over so that Pat does the stroking and Sam does the feedback of what's pleasurable and how it feels.

If you want to try this exercise, remember at this stage to avoid direct sexual contact. The goal is to experience touch and feedback. There is no demand for intercourse or orgasm so no fear of failure. Often this exercise increases affection between couples and each person can learn to recognize responsive areas of the body, feeling released to experiment with these rather than feeling an obligation to proceed automatically to what has previously been rather unsatisfactory intercourse or failure and resentment.

The next stage involves light stimulation of the genitals, still with no demand for intercourse. Pat and Sam use hand riding to guide the giver into learning what pleases the receiver. Mutual touching like this can lead to learning that arousal waxes and wanes so that it is not necessary to conclude that loss of arousal means failure.

The next stage can progress to stimulation to orgasm with each receiving partner telling the other how to make the stimulation arousing. If this is successful, then the groundwork has been laid for you to continue to explore sexual responsiveness in yourself and your partner as it pleases you both.

If this exercise elicits negative rather than pleasurable responses and talking over and practising the experience fails to identify ways in which it can be made more enjoyable, the problem may reside more in other aspects of the relationship or in more general anxiety or mood problems. These may need to be discussed with your doctor.

Don't give up. The drive for affection, intimacy and sex will still be around, even if buried under a lot of other problems to do with adjusting to your disability. Once you have decided it is time to explore it again, you can experiment in some of these ways to enhance your self-esteem and your whole quality of life.

11

Understanding phantom sensations

Phantom body parts

After amputation there is an almost universal sensation of the missing body part still being present, and sometimes it can be very painful. Almost everyone experiences a phantom limb for a short period. It is not just the amputation of arms and legs that can result in phantom body parts – some people have the sensation that their breasts or bladders still exist after their removal because of cancer. Phantom sensations can occur after other injuries too.

Brachial plexus avulsion

Gary had a motorcycle accident in which he collided with a car at high speed. A few days later he became aware that his right arm was not only useless but extremely painful. If he touched his hand he could feel nothing, but the hand itself seemed to be crushed in a vice with the finger nails digging into his palm. In addition he had periodic electric shock sensations from his neck to his hand which caused him to hunch forward. His arm was paralysed and completely numb but was exceedingly painful.

This condition is a consequence of brachial plexus avulsion. 'Brachial' means to do with the arm, a 'plexus' is a collection of nerves and 'avulsion' in this case means torn out of the spinal cord. As the car crashed into Gary's bike, he was flung off into the road but was still gripping the handlebars to try and steer out of the way. The energy of the sudden acceleration of his body forced apart his hand and his neck at the area where the nerves that operate the functions of his arm and hand leave the spinal cord.

So, Gary has an arm that is disconnected from its pathway between the brain and the hand, and the experiences that he now feels inside his hand are those of a phantom limb. Some people with this condition choose to have the arm amputated, but that normally makes no difference to the experience of pain because these sensations are not arising from the hand itself.

Spinal cord injury

A similar situation can arise after spinal cord injury, in which once again the body parts below the level of the break in the central nerve column are paralysed and unable to feel. Some people then experience strange sensations in their 'absent' areas such as tingling, burning or stabbing pains as if they are being attacked with hot knives or needles. They may also be aware that their limbs appear to be moving spontaneously although watching them produces a curious 'mismatch' between the sensation of movement and the appearance of complete immobility.

Eva, an ex-drug addict, who fell from a bridge five years ago and was paralysed as a result of her injuries, complained of these sensations, and she thought it most disconcerting to feel her legs move without any intention from her but to find that she was quite unable to get them to obey her when she tried to test out her ability to walk again. She asked for counselling, since she thought this was happening because she had not adjusted to her disability and a nurse had told her she was 'in denial'. Some people, like this nurse, believe these sensations occur because the brain refuses to change and adapt to the loss of functioning limbs. They may believe it is down to 'wishful thinking' and a 'desire to be normal'.

However, there is little evidence for this, and more recent scientific explanations imply that it is actually because the brain does change that phantom limbs present a problem.

Yasmin suddenly became very ill with a form of meningitis that causes blood poisoning. By the time she arrived in hospital she was already unconscious and one hand had been severely damaged by lack of circulation. Attempts to save her limb were unsuccessful and she had to have an amputation of her right arm below the elbow (a transradial amputation).

When she recovered, Yasmin immediately felt a great deal of pain as if the injured arm was still present. She felt very distressed about this but the doctors tried to reassure her that the pain would lessen in time. As the months went on she found this was not true and she struggled to cope with her disability as well as the prospect of learning to use an artificial limb – a prosthesis.

The homunculus and cortical remapping

To understand these sensations we need to look closely at some of the structures of the brain and at how the parts of the body are each mapped on to the cortex – the outer greyish layer of the brain. The brain itself is not sensitive to pain, so it is possible to stimulate bits of it systematically while people are undergoing brain surgery for other reasons and while they are conscious and can describe what they experience. Fascinating discoveries were made in this way by Wilder Penfield – a neurosurgeon working in the 1940s and 1950s. He found a strip of brain tissue towards the front of the brain on either side of the midline that corresponded to the various parts of the body, and as he stimulated different areas within it, the subjects reported feeling sensations in different body regions. Near the top of the brain he found the genital area represented and next to this he found stimulation produced sensations in the feet.

Further down this strip he found small areas representing the upper body and shoulders followed by a large area representing the hands. Next to this he found the lower face and lips. These took up a larger brain area than their actual size compared to the rest of the body because they are complex structures capable of very fine sensations and movements. They therefore have many more nerve connections. He called the figure that appeared the 'homunculus' or 'little man'. This is because it is very short, since the legs and trunk have relatively small areas of cortex devoted to them. The part of the brain that receives sensation from the body is the sensory cortex, and just in front of it is a similar strip involved in movement called the motor cortex.

There is some evidence that when a body part is lost, the nearest sensory cortex areas tend to take over the area belonging to the lost limb. For example, when a hand is amputated, the cells from the sensory cortex area belonging to the face may move into the area corresponding to the lost hand. This can mean that when the face is touched, nerve signals are sent to the sensory cortex area which now belongs to the face *and* the lost hand. There are lots of studies that demonstrate this, though it is not true of every person who has an arm amputation. We do not know why this is the case.

Sometimes, after amputation, people are not aware of it themselves until some fascinated doctor comes along and tries experimenting. This happened to Yasmin when she attended the limb-fitting clinic one morning to see about her artificial arm. After she had talked to the doctor for a while he asked a strange question.

Yasmin's experience

Doctor: Yasmin, would you mind if I stroke the right side of your face with this cotton bud?

Yasmin (somewhat surprised): OK.

Doctor: Can you tell me exactly what you feel when I do that?

Yasmin: I can feel you touching my face.

Doctor: Can you feel anything else? Do you feel me touching you anywhere else?

Yasmin: Well, I wasn't sure about this as I can't understand it but I seem to feel touch sensations in my absent hand.

Doctor: That's very good and just what I was looking for. Can you tell precisely which parts of your hand are stimulated when I touch different areas on your face?

Yasmin: When you touch my cheek, I think I can feel it in my thumb and my lips seem to be associated with my first two fingers. It feels very weird. Please stop.

Other people with high arm (transhumeral) amputations might experience something similar if they touch the cut end of the limb. The fingers appear to be nestling inside the stump (residual limb). This is because the area of the sensory cortex next to the hand on the other side from the face is the shoulder. Again it seems the sensory cells have moved into the 'empty' area left when the arm was cut off.

What happens with lower limbs?

Even more strange, though easier to understand now we have this much information, is Josef's complaint that he can feel pain in his phantom foot when he stands at the toilet to urinate. He suffered an amputation from an accident at work and has quite a lot of tingling in his phantom leg. Mostly he copes with this but finds it gets particularly bad when he goes to the toilet. It has also affected his sex life because he is afraid the strange sensations in his foot will increase if his genital area is stimulated. He saw a copy of the picture of the homunculus and could see that the genital area (relatively large) was right next to where his foot should have been, and he realized that the sensory nerve cells had spread out to invade his foot area.

This theory of changing areas in the sensory cortex is called remapping, and it is thought to explain some of the strange experiences of phantom limbs. It is also thought to be at least a partial explanation for pain in the phantom.

Remapping – sprouts or masks?

There are at least two theories doing the rounds at the moment as to how remapping occurs. Does the brain produce new sprouts of nerve connections? This could be one explanation but it is generally thought the central nervous system can't grow again in the way that other body tissues can. If it could, people would eventually recover from serious brain injury, which doesn't seem to be the case.

Alternatively, maybe the connections were there all the time and have become 'unmasked' by the loss of information coming back to the brain from the missing limb. Perhaps some of the brain started out with much less specialized connections when it belonged to a newborn baby and the connections became more specific as that baby grew up. This would allow the brain to make the most useful links as the child developed and to leave some in reserve so as to revise its ideas if something abnormal happened along the way. Then the brain does its best to fill the gap by recruiting these reserves.

It appears that if there is no input from the limb, this does not stop the nerve networks in the brain from generating messages to the missing limb or other body part. These messages give the sensation that the limb is present though it may not always be quite the right size or length. This process will continue throughout life after the limb has been amputated or, as we have seen, has been disconnected from its pathway to the cortex by spinal cord injury or brachial plexus avulsion or damage.

Movement and paralysis in phantom limbs

The situation with movement of body parts is similar but more complex, involving the integration of messages from several different brain areas. The motor cortex also contains a map of the body, but this time its purpose is to send messages to the muscles rather than to receive messages back from the body. Movements appear to happen when the motor cortex sends messages to the limbs. This seems to be what happens to Eva who feels movement in her paralysed legs, although the messages never actually arrive.

When Yasmin decides to take a drink using her left hand, the brain areas controlling her left arm will send a complex message to the muscles.

However, Yasmin was always right handed so it is likely that she will try and pick up her cup with her right hand. Her motor cortex will still send the command and the message will be received by other brain areas responsible for co-ordinating the movement. Of course it cannot reach the muscles of her right hand, but it will appear that the phantom arm is now moving. Should Yasmin drop the cup from her left hand, her right phantom arm might try very hard to help her catch it – just as it would have done before the accident.

Phantom pain

Gary and Yasmin both had painful phantom experiences for which normal pain killers were not very effective. Quite a lot of people (in fact almost 85 per cent in one recent survey) experience pain in their phantom limbs. Phantom pain sometimes decreases or disappears completely after a few months but for some people the pain can last much longer – in fact it may never go away. Or it might get better with time, only to recur if there is a further injury to the residual limb.

David was a landscape gardener who had a left transtibial (lower leg) amputation as a young man because of a football injury when he was a teenager. He managed extremely well with his artificial leg without any apparent disability. He never suffered from phantom pain but some 30 years later he was repairing a fence when a large concrete post snapped in half and fell on his legs just at the end of his stump (residual limb). David immediately felt pain in his missing ankle and foot which he had never experienced since the day after his leg had been amputated. Fortunately it soon went away.

Causes of phantom pain – psyche or soma?

In the past, pain was considered to be either 'psychogenic' (caused by emotional problems or all in the mind – the *psyche*) or 'organic' (caused by an injury in the body – the *soma*). Phantom pain, or any pain that cannot be explained by current knowledge of anatomy, is often discounted as 'psychosomatic' – that is, more in the mind than the body, perhaps the 'denial' that the nurse mentioned earlier. However, other researchers have not found any evidence to back this up. Rather it seems that psychological factors such as emotional distress can be a *reaction* to pain.

There are several theories that attempt to explain the cause of phantom pain. After the nerve endings have been cut during the amputation, they will attempt to grow again to join back together. Gradually little tendrils of nerve fibres will sprout and, because they have nothing to join up with, clumps of nerve endings will tangle together and cause 'neuromas'. These can become inflamed and irritated, and when this happens they send nerve signals back to the brain, which it interprets as pain. An operation to remove the neuroma can be successful although perhaps only temporarily, since the situation sometimes continues to occur each time the nerve is cut.

Other theories might be involved in remapping, as we have seen in Yasmin's case. There are pathways from the body to the sensory cortex that are apparently specific for the kind of information they carry – touch follows touch pathways and itch follows itch pathways. Pain follows complex pathways. It seems as if the nerve fibres might have become 'cross-wired', with touch fibres becoming attached to pain fibres as the face area spread out to fill the 'empty' hand area.

Pain gates

Then again, there is the theoretical role of gate control in perceiving and regulating pain. This theory developed from work in the 1960s by two scientists who described relays or 'gates' up the spine into the brain that evaluate the type of information that is travelling up the nerve pathways. They open or close to change its 'volume' depending on how serious it seems to be. This is why you only feel a small amount of pain when you prick your finger, and a larger amount of pain when you burn yourself. Pain exists to stop us from harming our bodies. However, when pain goes on for a long time (chronic pain), it has lost the 'emergency' message and the gates seem to be stuck in open mode. Chronic pain also changes the way the nerve pathways behave so they may become super-sensitive, often with changes in the chemical soup in which they function.

Abnormal chemicals irritate the nerve fibres and keep them constantly firing in irregular ways. These signals are also interpreted as pain by the time they reach the brain. Sometimes this situation appears to get worse with time and the nerves seem to get ever more sensitive. Less and less stimulation is needed to irritate them – sometimes even light touch will seem like excruciating pain. This process has acquired a very apt description: it is known as 'wind up'.

Another theory to explain phantom pain involves the concept that there is a specific 'memory' for pain. This will occur when the phantom limb feels the pain of the condition or accident that caused the amputation. Some pain experts have shown that a large proportion of people with phantom pain will describe it in the same terms as the pain they experienced in the body part before amputation. However, this does not apply to everyone and some people complain of phantom pain in a limb that was not painful before amputation. This certainly is a mystery. In this case it may be that nerve damage occurred during the operation itself and that this has been stored as the last memory the sensory cortex has about the limb.

Easier to understand but extremely frustrating is the continued experience of the very pain the amputation was performed to cure.

Debbie suffered from a painful bunion on her right foot. She was a model and needed to be able to walk as comfortably as possible down the catwalk in many different shoe styles. She had an operation but it was complicated by a main blood vessel being damaged by mistake. Amputation below the knee had to be performed because it became clear that there was no chance of saving the limb. During her rehabilitation, Debbie was most distressed to find that not only did she now have to contend with an artificial leg but she could still feel the pain of her bunion in her phantom limb.

It seems though that there will be a 'psyche' (emotional) component to all 'somatic' (physical) problems. To say the least, pain is an unpleasant experience, and it can be accompanied by mood changes such as anxiety and depression and by behavioural effects such as avoiding previously important activities. This can lead to loss of relationships, work and financial status. All these form a large psychological contribution and add to the stress that we have considered in previous chapters.

Stress is known to help the gates stay open. It can be caused by normal everyday difficulties like work or family concerns, or even by the pain itself. This can heighten awareness of phantom pain and end up in a vicious circle. Anxiety and depression make the management of chronic pain more difficult so it is very important to try to reduce or prevent these mood problems getting in the way. Post-traumatic stress disorder is common in people who have suffered amputation as a result of some horrific event and needs to be treated before phantom pain can be effectively dealt with.

Treatments for phantom pain – some initial ideas

Treatment of phantom pain poses a difficulty because traditional pain management programmes do not often take account of its special characteristics. A survey by a US doctor interested in the problems experienced by soldiers injured in wars identified 68 treatment methods in use in the USA. Dr Sherman found that most appeared to be only temporarily effective and only a very small number were considered moderately successful.

He did show that treatments aimed at reducing muscle tension significantly improved the cramping that is characteristic of phantom pain. This would indicate that treatments based on relaxation would have an effect. Further, he found that when the residual limb felt cool or cold, the intensity of burning, throbbing and tingling descriptions of phantom pain increased. Treatments based on increasing blood flow either with medical procedures or by biofeedback or imagery training have been shown to improve this aspect. Chapter 12 describes in more detail how these suggestions can be used. There are other treatments as well, which might be helpful in your particular case.

First it may be necessary to assess the type of pain you have and whether it has a pattern throughout the day. Have a look at the form below to see if one like it will help you record important aspects of your pain (Table 11.1). You may need to record your experience for several days to see if a pattern emerges. Then, when you try some of the techniques in the next chapter, you can note their effect and build up some evidence of what works for you.

Words most commonly chosen to describe the pain are 'burning', 'throbbing', 'shooting', 'stabbing', 'sharp', 'tingling' and 'crushing', but others may apply to you.

Table 11.1 Pain assessment chart

Date:

	No pain										Worst pain
Did you have difficulty sleeping?	0	1	2	3	4	5	6	7	8	9	10
Pain level this morning	0	1	2	3	4	5	6	7	8	9	10
Pain level this afternoon	0	1	2	3	4	5	6	7	8	9	10
Pain level this evening	0	1	2	3	4	5	6	7	8	9	10
Pain level after self-treatment	0	1	2	3	4	5	6	7	8	9	10

What was the pain like? Tick as applicable. Add any other descriptions that apply. Add up your score if you want to

	Mild (scores 1)	Moderate (scores 2)	Severe (scores 3)
Burning			
Throbbing			
Shooting			
Stabbing			
Sharp			
Tingling			
Crushing			

12

Treatments for phantom sensations

As we saw in the previous chapter, Dr Sherman recorded many different treatments for phantom discomfort and none seemed very effective in the long term. Pain medications may help if taken at the correct times and dosages but there are usually side effects, which may reduce your energy or concentration and prevent best levels of activity. You may have been given drugs to calm down shooting, electrical sensations. These are often effective but, unfortunately, the drugs are not 'smart' enough to target just the abnormal nerves so all the body systems are slowed, including the brain. You may feel drowsy and dizzy and your doctor will have to adjust the dose so that you get the best pain relief with the minimum of side effects, or you may have to give them up. Then it is best to consider the self-management approach.

Medical versus personal control

Medical control may involve:

Many consultations
Every one different
Diagnostic confusion
Interventions not successful
Control given away
Anger or frustration
Loss of confidence or hope.

Personal control may involve:

Progress
Exercise
Relaxation
Seizing back control
Own goals
Negative thoughts challenged
Achievement
Life improvement.

The second list might seem more inviting after a while.

Mirrors and movements

One of the ways in which you might try to gain personal control of your phantom discomfort is to use a mirror box.

In Chapter 11 we learned that some explanations for the phenomena of phantom sensations seem to involve the confusion the brain experiences between the image of the body as it is represented in the cortex and its actual appearance in reality. Dr Ramachandran, author of lots of fascinating facts in his book *Phantoms in the Brain*, describes some very interesting early experiments involving using a mirror image of the intact limb to 'trick' the brain into believing the amputated limb has suddenly reappeared. A number of studies have now been carried out using this approach and the results are able to help us understand a bit better what is happening.

Frank broke his right wrist but the injury deteriorated and nerve damage occurred. This resulted in a condition known as complex regional pain syndrome, and Frank requested an amputation. Afterwards, he was unable to move his phantom arm, which was still painful. He decided to try using a mirror box, which was just a cardboard box with an open top and two holes in which he attached a mirror lying horizontally. Frank inserted his left (intact) arm in the box in front of the mirror and then he attempted to place his phantom arm behind the mirror. By moving the intact limb until its reflection is on top of where the phantom limb appears to be, the brain 'perceives' the absent limb as if it were completing the circuit with its special portion of the sensory and motor cortex.

However, more recent research has taught us that it is not just the appearance of the missing limb in the mirror that helps the pain. The best results come from using the mirror to 'teach' the phantom limb to move and thus to feed back movement sensations to the right parts of the brain. If the intact limb performs some action like clapping, the phantom can join in so the movement is symmetrical. Then it appears that both the normal limb and the phantom limb are moving. Frank found that this overrode the paralysis present in his phantom limb and enabled him to move it into a more comfortable position. This reduced his pain temporarily, and with daily practice he was able to gain longer periods without so much discomfort.

Other studies with a taller box to help people with leg amputations have shown similar results. It may be worth your experimenting yourself. You can try it if you have a mirror door on a cupboard or a free standing tall mirror. Put your intact leg in front of the mirror and encourage your phantom to join in 'behind' the mirror with some movements like moving your toes up and down while watching the reflection. See if over time your phantom limb gets better at this. With practice you might find that you can decrease the discomfort.

One of the best ways of helping some people with phantom pain involves encouraging them to use their artificial limbs as much as possible. The limb-fitting clinic will seem a strange territory to start with but gradually you will get used to the techniques that are used. A plaster cast will be made of your residual limb (stump) at one of your early appointments so that the limb-fitting staff (your prosthetist) can make a socket to fit your stump to which the artificial limb (prosthesis) will be attached. You will then work with the rehabilitation therapists to improve your use of the prosthesis. As we have already learned, giving the brain the information it expects back from the limb when it has issued a command helps to complete the circuit and reduces pain. Some people find that, as long as they are wearing the prosthesis, they don't feel pain although it might recur when they take it off at night. Then they need to use some of the techniques discussed below.

Relaxation and imagery for modifying sensation

You can try using relaxation and imagery to change the sensations in the phantom limb. This might be better for you if you have no move-ment in your limbs after spinal injury or if you want to try imagination to encourage the phantom to move. It depends on using the power of your concentration to produce sensations that reduce the intensity of your feelings of discomfort. You may prefer to review Chapter 9 on mindfulness and meditation. In fact this technique is one that has developed from meditation practices.

In this technique you use your attention in a focused way. It usually involves people experiencing a sense of deep relaxation with their range of attention becoming highly selective. Although you might think it is similar to hypnosis (and you are probably right), there is nothing magical about it. In a state of relaxation you can be no less in touch with the world around you than you are when watching an absorbing film or reading a gripping novel. You will notice the phone ringing or other people moving about but you won't necessarily want to break your attention away from the relaxation task. You remain in a mindful state, concentrating specifically on the sensations that you wish to develop – this is very similar to the tasks you learned in mind-fulness meditation.

The stages of learning deep relaxation

1 Induction procedure

The induction procedure involves deliberately asking a group of muscles to become tired by keeping them completely still in an unnatural position. Fixing your eyes on an object such as a light switch and not allowing them to move, is an example. Your eyes will tend to close naturally after a while and you may feel more relaxed.

2 Deepening procedure

You may want to think about becoming more relaxed by counting to four. Each number represents deeper relaxation. Or you may think about relaxing a little more each time you breathe out.

3 Imagery development

You may want to increase your body temperature if warmth is comforting, or reduce it if you prefer coolness. A characteristic of your phantom sensation may suggest an image that helps to reduce your discomfort. Images that you create for yourself, based on your own experience, will be the most useful.

Most people have an extraordinary ability to create sensations in their bodies if they concentrate enough. The body responds as if the conditions existed in reality, as if the outside temperature really had changed, or the cool fountain or clear mountain air or a gentle pink colour were really there. The skill is being able to conjure up the conditions in imagination.

4 Return to general awareness

You will achieve this as soon as you want by counting back from four to one again, or just concentrating on being more alert.

Perhaps your CBT therapist (if you have one) has a tape or an audio CD for you to listen to at home so that you can practise. Or you can buy one (see the Further reading section, p. 114).

Examples of images in deep relaxation

Here are some examples of how to develop images while using deep relaxation. The first part is the induction procedure but feel free to use any other relaxation technique, such as mindfulness and body scan, if you prefer. You will notice the sentences are repeated quite a lot. This can help to keep you concentrating on the sensation you are trying to develop, but if it gets irritating, just read through the passages a few times and then say the instructions to yourself in any way that feels right for you.

You will notice the instruction to 'let the process continue as far as you want' crops up very frequently. This is to remind you that you are always in control and you can always choose what is most comfortable for you.

Warning: deep relaxation requires fixed concentration. You will not be able to concentrate on anything else at the same time. Do not practise this while driving or attempting any task that requires your attention.

Deep relaxation with warm imagery

Settle back comfortably and make sure your head and neck are well supported. Focus your eyes on a spot directly ahead of you and try and keep your eyes still and the spot in focus. The more you try and keep your eyes still the more tired they feel and the more blurred the spot becomes...Notice the sensations of tiredness and heaviness in your eyes and notice that the more tired and heavy your eyes feel the more relaxed you become all over...Concentrate on the feelings of tiredness and heaviness in your eyes and the feelings of relaxation in the rest of your body...Let those feelings develop...Notice that the more tired your eyes become the more difficult it is to keep them open...Notice how heavy your eyelids are feeling and how difficult it has become to keep the spot in focus and your eyes still...Just let those feelings develop, the feelings of tiredness and heaviness in your eyes and the feeling of relaxation all over your body...Notice that as you need to blink more it becomes more difficult to keep your eyes open...When your eyes feel so heavy that it is too difficult to keep them open any longer just let them close and focus on the feelings of relaxation and relief. Notice that as your eyes close you feel heavier and relaxed all over. Just let those feelings develop, concentrating on letting relaxation and heaviness develop all over your body, the more relaxed and heavy you become the more comfortable you feel...Just concentrate on the thought, 'I feel comfortable and relaxed...' Each time you breathe out, think about letting go and relaxing a bit further and a bit further. Each time you breathe out relax a little more...

Now think about increasing relaxation even further by counting to four, with each number becoming even more relaxed and comfortable. Number one, very relaxed and comfortable. Number two, even more relaxed and comfortable. Number three, more and more relaxed and comfortable, and number four, very relaxed and comfortable now.

Just concentrate on the feelings of comfort and relaxation and let the process continue as far as you like...Focus on the thought, 'My body feels comfortable and relaxed.'

Now imagine sitting by a warm fire. Notice the heat of the fire and concentrate on the feelings of warmth in your skin that develop in response to the heat of the fire. Notice your skin becoming warmer and warmer, and the warmer your skin feels the more comfortable and relaxed you become...Focus on the thought, 'My skin feels warm,' and let the process continue as far as you want...Or imagine lying in a bath of warm water. Notice the heat of the water and concentrate on the feelings of warmth that develop in your skin in response to the heat of the water. Let the feelings of warmth increase, and the warmer your skin feels the more comfortable and relaxed you become...Concentrate on the thought, 'My skin feels warm,' and let the process continue as far as you want...Or imagine lying in the sun. Concentrate on the feelings of heat and notice how warm your skin feels in response to the heat of the sun. Concentrate on increasing the feelings of warmth in your skin, and the warmer your skin feels, the more comfortable and relaxed you feel. Focus on the thought, 'My skin feels warm,' and let the process continue as far as you want...

Now think about your remaining areas of discomfort and notice that the more warm and relaxed you feel, the more your areas of discomfort will decrease. Imagine your areas of discomfort becoming smaller and smaller and let the process continue as far as you want... Notice your areas of discomfort decreasing in size and let the process continue so that when you want to finish you can take the decreased areas of discomfort away with you. Let them continue to get smaller and smaller as far as you like...Concentrate on the sense of control that you have over your areas of discomfort. The more comfortable and relaxed you become, the smaller your remaining areas of discomfort can grow... Focus on the thought, 'My body feels comfortable and relaxed...' Just let the feelings of comfort and relaxation take the place of discomfort and tension. Notice that the more comfortable and relaxed you feel, the smaller your areas of discomfort will become. When you finish you can take these decreased areas of discomfort away with you. Focus on the thought, 'My body feels comfortable and relaxed.'

Think about the key words 'relax' and 'warm'. Whenever you think about the word 'relax', think about becoming relaxed and comfortable, and when you think about the word 'warm', think about increasing feelings of warmth and comfort taking the place of feelings of burning and discomfort. Use the key words 'relax' and 'warm' to produce feelings of relief from discomfort. Let the process continue as far as you want, so that when you want to finish you can take the feelings of warmth away with you and let them disperse any feelings of tension and discomfort.

When you want to end your session, think about counting back from four to one again, and with each number become more alert and awake. Think about number four, becoming more alert and at number three, more alert. At number two, much more alert and at number one quite alert and awake, feeling refreshed and comfortable, relaxed and in control.

Deep relaxation with cool imagery

If you would prefer cool imagery, try this variation. The technique is pretty similar to the warm one. Many people favour warm sensations even if they have burning pain, but the choice is yours.

Start with the same induction as before, up to the point where you have counted from one to four to deepen the relaxation.

Now think about what it feels like to be in a cool shower. Think about the sensations of coolness, of being refreshed, cool and comfortable. Let your skin react to the feelings of coolness and comfort from the cool water of the shower. Imagine being in the shower and turning the temperature of the water until it becomes cool and comforting and refreshing. Just imagine adjusting the temperature of the shower until it is so cool and refreshing that you feel very comfortable...Focus on the thought, 'My skin feels cool and comfortable...' Think about removing all sensations of heat and tension and letting the cool, comfortable temperature of the water take their place. Turn the temperature of the water until the skin feels as cool and comfortable as you want... Let the process continue until you feel cool and comfortable all over, and the more cool and refreshed you feel, the more comfortable and relaxed you become...Focus on the thought, 'My skin feels cool and comfortable.'

Now think about being in a place where there is a cool breeze. Imagine what it's like to be in a cool breeze on a hot day. Imagine the feelings of the cool breeze on your skin, imagine the cool breeze taking away the feelings of heat and burning from your skin. Just let the cool breeze cool your skin until it feels comfortable...Just let the process continue as far as you want...Think about the coolness taking away the feelings of burning and heat and tension, and the more cool your skin feels the more comfortable and relaxed you feel...Focus on the thought, 'My skin feels cool and comfortable.'

Now think about drinking a glass of cool drink on a very hot day. Imagine the sensations of coolness and refreshment as you drink the glass of cool water. Let the feelings of coolness and refreshment take the place of feelings of heat and burning and tension...Think about the effect of the glass of cool water in cooling you, refreshing you and taking away the feelings of burning and discomfort...Focus on the thought, 'My body feels cool and comfortable...' Let the feelings of coolness take the place of feelings of burning and tension and discomfort...Let the process continue until you feel as comfortable as you want. Now think about your remaining areas of discomfort and notice that the more cool and relaxed you feel, the more your areas of discomfort will decrease. Imagine your areas of discomfort becoming smaller and smaller and let the process continue as far as you want... Notice your areas of discomfort decreasing in size and let the process continue. Let them continue to get smaller and smaller as far as you like...Concentrate on the sense of control that you have over your areas of discomfort. The more comfortable and relaxed you become, the smaller your remaining areas of discomfort can grow...Let the process continue until your areas of discomfort are as small as you like and when you want to finish you can take these much reduced areas away with you...Concentrate on increasing the feelings of comfort and relaxation and letting these feelings take the place of feelings of discomfort and tension. Just let the process continue...Focus on the thought, 'My body feels cool and comfortable, and let the feelings of coolness continue to develop until there are no feelings of burning or heat or discomfort. The feelings of coolness and comfort have taken their place. Let the process continue as far as you want, so that when you finish you can take the sensations of coolness and comfort away with you. Focus on the thought, 'I feel cool and comfortable.' The more relaxed you become, the cooler and more comfortable you can feel.

Think about the key words 'relax' and 'cool'. Whenever you think about the word 'relax', think about becoming relaxed and comfortable with no tension, and when you think about the word 'cool', think about turning down any feelings of heat and burning and discomfort. The word 'cool' can conjure up for you the feelings of coolness, refreshment and comfort to take the place of feelings of heat and burning and discomfort. Use the key words 'relax' and 'cool' to bring about these feelings of relief from tension and burning and discomfort...Let the process continue as far as you want, so that when you want to finish you can take the feelings of coolness away with you and use them to disperse any feelings of heat and burning and discomfort.

When you want to end your session think about counting back from four to one again, becoming more alert and awake with each number. Think about number four, becoming more alert and at number three, more alert. At number two, much more alert and at number one quite alert and awake, feeling refreshed and cool, relaxed and in control.

Josef, who experienced tingling sensations in his phantom foot while standing at the toilet, tried these techniques and found he could change the temperature in his foot so that the tingling stopped. He used this strategy before he attempted to restore his sexual relationship with his wife and quickly gained confidence.

Other images

Here are some other images you might want to consider. The words which seemed to be most often changed by this technique are 'burning', 'throbbing', 'shooting', 'stabbing', 'sharp', 'tingling' and 'cramping'.

If your discomfort is a burning pain imagine it as a candle. Focus your attention on the flame of the candle and watch it melt the wax. Imagine your discomfort like the wax, melting away as the candle burns down, the areas of discomfort becoming smaller and shorter.

Or imagine watching a parade along a street. The procession is headed by a marching band, beating time with a big bass drum. Watch the procession move further and further down the street, the bass drum keeping pace with your throbbing pain and getting fainter as the band moves off into the distance. As the drum gets further away, your throbbing pain gets fainter and fainter. Let the process continue as far as you want.

Imagine a beautiful, white, sandy beach which you are travelling along. The waves are rushing in and out as the tide moves inwards and then outwards. As the waves come in, picture them taking hold of your shooting pain, then as they move out they carry your pain away with them. Each wave takes the pain further away from your body, leaving it refreshed and comfortable.

If your areas of discomfort feel stabbing and sharp as if caused by a knife or hot needle, imagine them turning into ice and slowly melting away, taking with them the sharp or stabbing feeling...Imagine the sensations of coldness taking the place of the discomfort as the sensations melt away with the ice.

Or imagine a tingling feeling as the colour red. Take a deep breath and as you breathe out feel the red fading to a lighter red, then an even lighter red and then finally fading completely so there is no colour left and the tingling subsides.

Now concentrate on the sensations you would experience if you were lying in a light sunny field. Feel the light penetrating your body and easing away cramping discomfort. As the light penetrates, feel it begin to stretch out the cramping discomfort, as though you are unwinding and stretching out a length of elastic...Attend to the feelings of stretching and unwinding. The more you stretch the more comfortable you feel... let the process continue as far as you like.

These are a few suggestions but even better would be images that you invent for yourself, depending on what your areas of discomfort feel they want to do.

Use the record form in the previous chapter to check your progress if you like (see Table 11.1).

13

Conclusion: turn things out for the best

This is the point in this book at which you now need to take over and decide if you have found something useful for your particular circumstances. The chapters have been based on the strategies that have proved helpful for people with disabilities to build lasting acceptance and self-esteem, so perhaps at least some of the ideas will be of use to you too. Of course, it all takes practice. ACT is about commitment and your real work now is to find your own way of dealing with your remaining difficulties. Acquiring a disability is undoubtedly a life-changing event but it doesn't have to be a disaster that lays waste to all your values and aspirations.

We have looked at how you can identify and challenge thoughts that are demoralizing and overwhelming so that they lead to avoidance of valuable activities, and we have discussed ways in which you can explore your thoughts, mood states and responses. We have paid some attention to the effects of stress, including post-traumatic stress disorder, which commonly accompanies illnesses and accidents that result in lasting disability. Some suggestions have been relaxation, mindful meditation and imagery, particularly for the mysterious experience of phantom sensations.

Take control of what you want

Setting goals is fundamental to understanding how to get from where you are now to where you would like to be, and we have looked at some ways to keep you motivated to move forward. Also, we have explored communication styles that should enable you to get the help you want without being patronized or overburdened. This applies to all kinds of relationships from dealing with the health, local authority and legal professions to enjoying greater intimacy with your partner. So now it's your turn to decide on your life values and on your goals for the next stage of your life and to take control of your future. It will not be without its challenges but you can take a breathing space whenever you think it is all too worrying and difficult. Remember the power of the breath of life in helping to refocus and in letting the internal barriers pass along as events in the mind rather than reality.

You might be interested in how things turned out for the characters who have acted as our models in the situations we have explored. Clive, Leroy, Yasmin and Frank all had pain as well as disability and entered further pain management programmes before returning to work. Anil also had this problem and was unable to go back to his job, but he was very keen on DIY projects. He needed quite frequent 'top ups' to remind him about pacing his target achievements but eventually developed a good system with Rena to minimize his time in bed. He was often called upon to talk about his experience to newly injured people and learned to have good self-esteem because he could see he was of help. Debbie retrained as a designer for the fashion industry and found her bunion pain was not so intrusive while she was concentrating on her work. She practised relaxation and imagery to help her sleep if she was disturbed by pain at night. Gary changed his job to a better paid one, took up chess and learned to drive a car instead of a motor bike. Eva and Omar both work with young people to help them to avoid the effects of disengagement, drug use, gun crime and involvement with terrorism.

Maria and Ella met at a wheelchair clinic and encouraged each other to go out socially and volunteer for community projects. Anne, Sheena and Mary all joined assertiveness groups to build up their self-confidence, and Alex found a life partner and had two children. His parents were so pleased about this that they stopped remarking on his disability and began to admire his family skills instead, especially when his sister disappointed them by divorcing her husband.

Josef continued to learn about managing his prosthesis, and Sally grew in confidence with her boyfriend so that she started to believe that he loved a lot of things about her, including her 'little leg'. She was initially very challenging to her limb-fitting centre by complaining about most aspects of the service she received but she joined an action group and is gradually helping the staff improve their expectations of people's needs for modern prosthetic components using her newly found assertive manner.

As you might expect, Joshua required extensive CBT to deal with his core beliefs but eventually he became good enough at it to dispense with his internalized mother and began to train as a therapist himself. He was particularly good at helping people fill in their goal attainment forms!

All these people were able to make use of the techniques we have explored and build on them. Some used the further resources at the end of this book (see pp.112–13), so these resources might help you too.

Remember these are all based on real people. They improved their quality of life so you can too. If you get stuck, try and think about the form your barrier is taking and review the relevant section to overcome it or identify what further help you need.

Best of luck!

Useful addresses

Army Welfare Service
Tel.: 01722 436569
Website: www.army.mod.uk

Binley's Handbook of Patient Groups
Beechwood House
2–3 Commercial Way
Christy Close
Southfields
Basildon
Essex SS15 6EF
Tel.: 01268 495600
Website: www.binleys.com

British Limbless Ex-Servicemen's Association (BLESMA)
185–187 High Road
Chadwell Heath
Romford
Essex RM6 6NA
Tel.: 0208 590 1124
Website: www.blesma.org

Combat Stress
Tyrwhitt House
Oaklawn Road
Leatherhead
Surrey KT22 0BX
Tel.: 01372 841600
Website: www.combatstress.org.uk

Ministry of Defence
Website: www.mod.uk

National Association for Bikers with a Disability (NABD)
Unit 20, The Bridgewater Centre
Robson Avenue
Urmston
Manchester M41 7TE
Tel.: 0844 415 4849
Website: www.nabd.org.uk

NHS Direct
Tel.: 0845 4647
Website: www.nhsdirect.nhs.uk

Spinal Injuries Association
SIA House
2 Trueman Place
Oldbrook
Milton Keynes MK6 2HH
Tel.: 0800 980 0501 (freephone advice line 9.30 a.m. to 1 p.m./2 to
4.30 p.m., Monday to Friday)
Website: www.spinal.co.uk

Traumatic Brachial Plexus Injury Group
TBPI Group
1 Malvern Rise
Hadfield
Glossop SK13 1QW
Tel.: 01457 867140
Website: www.tbpiukgroup.homestead.com

Further reading

Christian, A. *Lower Limb Amputation: a guide to living a quality life*. Demos Medical Publishing, New York, 2005.

Cole, F., Macdonald, H., Carus, C. and Howden-Leach, H. *Overcoming Chronic Pain*. Robinson, London, 2005.

Dryden, W. *How to Accept Yourself*. Sheldon Press, London, 1999.

Greenberger, D. and Padesky, C. *Mind Over Mood*. Guildford Press, New York, 1995.

Kabat-Zinn, J. *Full Catastrophe Living: using the wisdom of your body and mind to face stress, pain, and illness*. (With audio compact discs.) Piatkus Books, London, 1996.

Kaufman, M., Silverberg, C. and Odette, F. *The Ultimate Guide to Sex and Disability*. Cleis Press, California, 2003.

Masters, W., Johnson, V. and Kolodny, R. *Sex and Human Loving*. Little, Brown, New York, 1988.

Ramachandran, V. and Blakeslee, S. *Phantoms in the Brain: human nature and the architecture of the mind*. Fourth Estate, London, 1999.

Sandowski, C. *Sexual Concerns When Illness or Disability Strikes*. Charles Thomas, Illinois, 1989.

Willson, R. and Branch, R. *Cognitive Behavioural Therapy for Dummies*. John Wiley, Chichester, 2006.

Index